THE
EVERYTHING®
DASH DIET COOKBOOK

Dear Reader,

In 2004, I was diagnosed with an inner-ear disorder called Meniere's disease. Rather than medication or surgery, my doctor prescribed a low-sodium DASH diet as my course of treatment. The idea that a change in diet could cure my ills seemed inconceivable at that point, but I did as instructed. I eliminated salt from my diet and modified my sodium intake to less than 1,500 mg per day.

Within weeks, I began noticing a change in my symptoms, and within months, the dizziness, deafness, and constant tinnitus I'd been experiencing for almost a year had virtually disappeared. It was the most miraculous physical transformation I'd ever experienced; *concrete proof of the power of diet.*

Whatever has brought you to the DASH diet, I am here to tell you: it works. Just as overly salted and heavily processed foods have the ability to harm your body, you have the power to help it heal, meal by healthy meal.

The DASH diet is intended to be a healthy eating plan for life, something to embrace and enjoy. I'm honored to join you on your journey to health, and wish you every happiness in the future.

Christy Ellingsworth

Welcome to the EVERYTHING® Series!

These handy, accessible books give you all you need to tackle a difficult project, gain a new hobby, comprehend a fascinating topic, prepare for an exam, or even brush up on something you learned back in school but have since forgotten.

You can choose to read an Everything® book from cover to cover or just pick out the information you want from our four useful boxes: e-questions, e-facts, e-alerts, and e-ssentials. We give you everything you need to know on the subject, but throw in a lot of fun stuff along the way, too.

We now have more than 400 Everything® books in print, spanning such wide-ranging categories as weddings, pregnancy, cooking, music instruction, foreign language, crafts, pets, New Age, and so much more. When you're done reading them all, you can finally say you know Everything®!

QUESTION

Answers to common questions

FACT

Important snippets of information

ALERT

Urgent warnings

ESSENTIAL

Quick handy tips

PUBLISHER Karen Cooper

MANAGING EDITOR, EVERYTHING® SERIES Lisa Laing

COPY CHIEF Casey Ebert

ACQUISITIONS EDITOR Brett Palana-Shanahan

DEVELOPMENT EDITOR Brett Palana-Shanahan

EDITORIAL ASSISTANT Matthew Kane

EVERYTHING® SERIES COVER DESIGNER Erin Alexander

LAYOUT DESIGNERS Erin Dawson, Jessica Faria, Michelle Roy Kelly, Elisabeth Lariviere

Visit the entire Everything® series at *www.everything.com*

THE EVERYTHING® DASH DIET COOKBOOK

Lower your blood pressure and lose weight—with 300 quick and easy recipes!

Christy Ellingsworth and Murdoc Khaleghi, MD

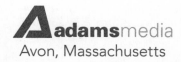

Avon, Massachusetts

To those who struggle with their health and want to be whole again; it's time.

An Everything® Series Book.
Everything® and everything.com® are registered trademarks of F+W Media, Inc.

Published by Adams Media, a division of F+W Media, Inc.
57 Littlefield Street, Avon, MA 02322 U.S.A.
www.adamsmedia.com

ISBN 10: 1-4405-4353-4
ISBN 13: 978-1-4405-4353-1
eISBN 10: 1-4405-4354-2
eISBN 13: 978-1-4405-4354-8

Printed in the United States of America.

10 9 8 7 6 5 4 3 2 1

Always follow safety and common-sense cooking protocol while using kitchen utensils, operating ovens and stoves, and handling uncooked food. If children are assisting in the preparation of any recipe, they should always be supervised by an adult.

This book is available at quantity discounts for bulk purchases.
For information, please call 1-800-289-0963.

Contents

Acknowledgments

For their love and support always, I thank my family. And to the Big Guy, although I may sometimes wonder out loud, I trust you know what you're doing.

—CE

You Have the Power to Change Your Life

THE DASH DIET, OR the Dietary Approaches to Stop Hypertension, is not just a diet. Quite simply, the DASH diet can change your life. Imagine if there was a medication that could significantly reduce your risk for heart disease, a stroke, cancer, with the only side effects being weight loss and improved energy. What would that be worth to you? Now imagine you could achieve such a dramatic change in your life without having to take any medication. You just have to eat, something you already do anyway. All you need to actively do is change some of the foods you eat.

You may then think the foods you have to change to would be very restrictive, like a lot of the diets out there. Again, the DASH diet is not just a diet; it's a way to change your life. The only way to permanently change your life is to do something you can do permanently. Therefore, the DASH diet was designed to be something that you could easily incorporate into your life. You do not need to shop at special grocery stores or go through some of the difficult transition periods of other diets; you just need to start adjusting your food patterns, one step at a time.

The basics of the diet are simple: Eat more fruits and vegetables, whole grains, and lean protein, and eat less saturated fats, salt, and sweets. The problem with leaving it at that is there are no actual guidelines as to how much of what you should eat. The DASH diet fixes that problem.

The DASH diet is not just an idea that someone came up with and hoped might work. It was scientifically developed based on many large studies at several prestigious government, university, and hospital research institutions. Its benefits have been repeatedly confirmed, and new benefits are always being discovered. The DASH diet has been repeatedly shown to improve many cholesterol and inflammatory biomarkers that are associated with risks for various diseases. You can easily see the impact on your own biomarkers through a service such as WellnessFX, and see the actual effects the DASH diet has on your own body.

For all these reasons, the DASH diet has been repeatedly rated as the overall best diet in the world by several organizations, including the *US News and World Report*. Unlike many diets that become a fad only to disappear as quickly as they became popular, the DASH diet's popularity has lasted for many years and is only growing.

The biggest challenge of the DASH diet is making the dietary transition. This book is your key to making that transition. In addition to giving you the guidelines for the amounts of various foods you should eat, we actually provide you the recipes so you can start right away with eating delicious foods that follow the DASH diet.

The knowledge and tools in this book can change your life. All you need to supply is the motivation. Since you are reading this book, you already have. Congratulations on taking that first essential step to making your life healthier.

—Murdoc Khaleghi, MD

Introduction

WHETHER YOU PICKED UP this book out of simple curiosity or dire need, *The Everything® DASH Diet Cookbook* is intended to make life on a low-sodium diet easy and pleasurable. For those new to the diet, DASH is an acronym for Dietary Approaches to Stop Hypertension. The DASH diet is a healthy, balanced eating plan low in sodium and rich in fruits, vegetables, whole grains, and low-fat dairy products. Meats, sweets, and nuts are all permitted, although added sugars and fats should be eaten in moderation.

A low-sodium DASH diet is often prescribed for those with serious medical conditions and has been shown to aid the body in healing by lowering blood pressure, reducing cholesterol, and promoting heart health and wellness in general. As with many sensible eating plans, it has the added bonus of promoting healthy weight loss and weight maintenance, and may also aid in the prevention of cancer, osteoporosis, and diabetes. In short, the DASH diet has the potential for helping millions of people live longer, healthier lives.

But in order to benefit, you must make the commitment! In practice, many fall short of dietary goals because of their impracticality. Modern lives are endlessly busy, and because of this, good eating often takes a backseat until a health crisis erupts. *The Everything® DASH Diet Cookbook* was written with this in mind. With more than 300 simple, inexpensive, and delicious recipes—all with 30 minutes or less of cooking time—there's no excuse not to make yourself and your health a priority.

On the DASH diet, you will be enjoying many of the same foods you've always eaten: fresh fruits and vegetables, low-fat dairy products, whole grains, beans, meats, even desserts. You will not feel deprived! But you will need to adapt. Salt-free living isn't easy, but it's worth it because *you're worth it!* Freeing yourself from the burden of bad health is a challenge to be taken to heart (pun intended).

The first step to starting the DASH diet is simple: Stop using salt. From there you'll need to stock a low-sodium pantry, seeking out products specifically created for a salt-free, low-sodium audience. It helps to purchase a small food-counts book until you're familiar with the sodium content of most common foods. You may want to keep it in your purse or pocket and consult it while shopping or dining out.

The good news is you can either buy or make everything you will need to live normally on the DASH diet. And as a low-sodium diet becomes more mainstream, companies are increasingly answering demand by expanding product lines, making salt-free cooking even easier and more convenient.

Use the recipes and information contained within this book to spark your own imagination. Wherever you live, seek out stores and scour for products that meet low-sodium criteria (140 mg or less per serving). Engage with the world around you, visiting local farms and farmers' markets, to buy the freshest and best produce, preferably organic whenever possible. New dishes will inevitably grow out of each season, and by incorporating the freshest ingredients, you'll be giving your body the best you possibly can. Outside of diet alone, explore every avenue at your disposal for healthy living. Join a gym, take an exercise class, or just go outside and take a walk, daily if possible. Look forward to spending time taking care of yourself.

A low-sodium diet is something you must commit to. You can't slack off and expect to make inroads. It can be hard, but don't give up. Your body will thank you! On those days when you feel as though you're simply treading water, remind yourself: you're in the pool! Those above you on the bleachers can see your progress, even when you can't. You may struggle with fatigue, but with daily practice you're building endurance, and ultimately, success.

CHAPTER 1

The DASH Diet

The DASH diet has become one of the most popular dietary lifestyles today. When many people hear the word "diet," they assume it is temporary. The DASH diet is not meant to be temporary though, it is designed to be a permanent lifestyle to make you healthier!

What Does DASH Mean?

DASH stands for Dietary Approaches to Stop Hypertension. Though the diet was created with a focus on hypertension, over the last decade it has been found to effect much more. The DASH diet has been shown to lower blood pressure, improve cholesterol, decrease the risk of many types of cancer, and even decrease the chance of kidney stones!

Show Me the Evidence

Unlike many dietary plans, the DASH diet has been put through rigorous scientific testing. It has been studied by the National Institute of Health, the premier governmental research organization, and at many prestigious universities and medical centers through multicenter trials. Though the DASH diet itself does not have strict controls, the studies enforced strict controls on what subjects were eating to ensure the reliability of the data. Ever since those initial studies, the DASH diet continues to be studied in terms of how it might affect other diseases. New benefits are constantly being discovered.

FACT

The DASH diet was originally formed with the goal of improving hypertension through diet. Since its formation, it has been found to have many other health benefits, from decreasing the risk of cancer to reducing the risk of heart attack and stroke.

Between all these benefits and how the DASH diet is designed to maximize compliance and sustainability, it is no wonder that the DASH diet is often considered the most popular diet among physicians and health organizations. In fact, the *US News and World Report* magazine has repeatedly ranked the DASH diet as the number one overall diet plan.

High Blood Pressure

Hypertension, or high blood pressure, was the initial focus of the diet because hypertension is known to be one of the largest killers in American society. In addition, it is considered a "silent" killer, because you do not feel the effects of high blood pressure for years until it actually causes a heart attack or stroke. These occur when plaques that build up in our arteries clog a blood vessel and do not allow blood and oxygen flow to our heart and brain, respectively. A heart attack can result in the heart not being able to pump blood to the rest of the body, and a stroke can result in your brain being unable to control your body. Ultimately, heart attacks and strokes are the leading causes of death in our society, and strokes are a major cause of paralysis in those who survive them. By reducing the formation of these plaques, you can reduce your risk of death and disability. To reduce these plaques, you need to understand what causes them and how your diet contributes to them.

ALERT

High blood pressure is considered one of the leading causes of death in developed nations, despite not feeling the effects of high blood pressure for years. For this reason, it is often called a "silent" killer.

Blood pressure is the pressure your blood exerts on the blood vessel, which is also the pressure used by your heart to push blood through your body. The higher your blood pressure, the more damage that occurs to your blood vessels, with these damaged areas forming plaques that can cause a heart attack and stroke. This damage builds up over many years, which again is why high blood pressure is known as a silent killer, doing its damage over the course of many years. In addition, the higher your blood pressure the harder your heart has to work; therefore, the more predisposed it becomes to failing. By controlling high blood pressure before it affects your body, you can successfully reduce your risk for a heart attack or stroke. Even more fortunately, no matter how long you may have had high blood pressure, you can still reduce your risk by acting on it now. In other words, it is never too late to help yourself.

Blood pressure is measured in millimeters of mercury or mmHg. There are actually two blood pressure measurements, the pressure exerted by your heart and blood when it is actively pumping or the *systolic* blood pressure, and the pressure exerted when the heart is not actively pumping or the *diastolic* blood pressure. Blood pressure measurements are displayed by showing the systolic blood pressure over the diastolic blood pressure. People who have a blood pressure greater than 140/90 mmHg are considered *hypertensives* or to have high blood pressure.

Does the Diet Work?

The DASH diet has consistently and repeatedly been shown to successfully reduce blood pressure. The general consensus is that people with normal blood pressure following the diet have a reduction of about 6 mmHg in their systolic blood pressure and 3 mmHg in their diastolic blood pressure. People with high blood pressure experience approximately twice this reduction in both systolic and diastolic blood pressures.

QUESTION

Is the DASH diet just another fad diet?
The DASH diet has been repeatedly studied by many prestigious institutions, and has been consistently shown to have many significant benefits to health. These effects have now been known for years and are repeatedly verified.

This sort of reduction can significantly reduce cardiovascular risk and is comparable to many blood pressure medications. Unlike costly blood pressure medications with their many deleterious side effects, the only side effects of the diet are improvement in blood pressure, cholesterol, cancer risk, and weight.

Why Does It Work?

The DASH diet is a sustainable lifestyle because it does not impose many of the strict restrictions that exist with many other diets. Rather than strict control of food or content choices, such as number of grams of fat, the DASH diet is primarily driven by guidelines to make smart food choices. This lack of severe restriction allows you to gradually transition to a DASH diet, and maintain that lifestyle once fully transitioned. Other diets often require a sudden change, and have such tight restrictions it is impossible to maintain the diet for a long period of time.

The goals of the DASH diet are to reduce your intake of substances that hurt your body, and substitute that intake with more healthful substances. For example, rather than consuming foods high in saturated fat, sodium, and sugars, you eat more foods low in fat and sodium and high in protein and complex carbohydrates. It also makes sure that you eat even these healthful foods in moderation and not in excess.

You Are What You Eat

To best understand how the DASH diet affects your body, all you need is a basic primer in digestive physiology. The body absorbs three substances in food: protein, carbohydrates, and fat. Protein is primarily used for muscle and other tissue generation, while carbohydrates and fat are primarily used for energy. The body uses carbohydrates initially for energy, and then when low on those easily usable carbohydrates, the body starts to break down fat for energy. In other words, carbohydrate intake initially gets stored as "fat." Often people consume more carbohydrates than their bodies can initially use. In that situation, the body produces a hormone called insulin, which stores the carbohydrates in your body, and some of those excess carbohydrates are converted to stored fat as well.

What Your Body Sees

Carbohydrates, protein, and fat all have a certain amount of energy, which is measured in calories. The average person typically uses just over 2,000 calories per day. Carbohydrates and protein each have 4 calories per gram, while fats have 9 calories per gram. In other words, fats have more than double the energy per gram than carbohydrates and protein. Therefore, ingesting more fats will quickly increase the number of calories you take in, and by consuming excess calories you increase the storage of fat. Though there are good types of fat, which will be discussed later, in general the more stored fat you have the worse that fat is, and therefore you want to decrease the amount of fat that is stored. Another way to decrease the storage of fat is to increase your activity, which will increase your energy consumption above the 2,000-calorie average. So by increasing your activity, you will consume less excess calories, and therefore store less fat.

Carbohydrates

Carbohydrates are the primary fuel for the body and have gotten a bad rap lately. Carbohydrates often get consumed in excess, causing an increase in the release of a hormone called *insulin*, which stores the carbohydrates as fat. Insulin spikes also make you feel fatigued and promote *insulin resistance*, a precursor for diabetes. Therefore, carbohydrates can be bad when too much enters the bloodstream at once but can appropriately fuel the body when consumed in moderation and with a steady release into the bloodstream. *Complex carbohydrates*, or carbohydrates that are linked together, are broken down more steadily when digested than *simple carbohydrates*, the types of sugars found in sweets, which do not have these same linkages. Simple carbohydrates enter the bloodstream all at once, giving you a sudden boost of energy or "sugar rush," which soon goes away. Like decreasing your weight, having a steady, moderate consumption of complex carbohydrates will improve your energy and offer many other health benefits.

Sodium

Sodium is the primary ingredient in the most common form of salt. When you eat salt, sodium gets absorbed into your bloodstream. This increases the concentration of sodium in your blood compared to other tissues in your body. By *osmosis*, or the tendency of fluid to follow particles in that fluid, fluid in tissues flow back into the bloodstream. The more fluid there is in your bloodstream, the greater the pressure that fluid exerts on your heart and blood vessels, or the higher your blood pressure. Putting it all together, ingesting more salt increases your blood pressure.

Fat and Cholesterol: The Good and the Bad

As mentioned previously, high blood pressure creates damage to your blood vessels, which causes the formation of plaques that can lead to heart disease and stroke. What further contributes to this damage is the buildup of cholesterol-filled clots in excessive amounts of fat and cholesterol. Interestingly, though, certain types of fat and cholesterol seem to actually decrease this plaque formation. If you were to get your cholesterol measured, it would be broken down into certain good types of cholesterol, the most common being *high-density lipoprotein (HDL) cholesterol*, and certain bad types of cholesterol, the most common being *low-density lipoprotein (LDL) cholesterol*. Generally, HDL cholesterol decreases plaque formation, and LDL cholesterol increases plaque formation. Actually, your physiology is far more complex than these two common lipoproteins, as they have many different subtypes, but to review them all would be a book in itself. It is still important to know and track all your numbers, though, and you can easily do this by signing up for a comprehensive testing service such as WellnessFX at their website, *www.wellnessfx.com*.

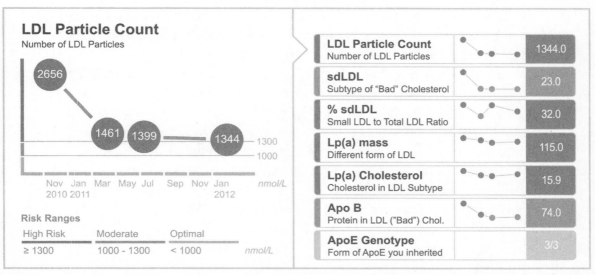

Printed with copyright permission courtesy of WellnessFX.

Saturated fats and trans fats, two unhealthy types of fats, typically lower your HDL cholesterol and increase your LDL cholesterol, therefore increasing plaque buildup. Unsaturated fats, such as monounsaturated omega-3 fatty acids, have been shown to have the opposite effect. In addition, while the bad fats and obesity have been shown to increase inflammation in the body—which is also associated with plaque buildup and other diseases such as cancer—these monounsaturated fatty acids have been shown to decrease inflammation. These unsaturated fats are most commonly found in fruits and vegetables in low concentrations, and fish in higher concentrations.

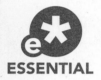

ESSENTIAL

Not all fat is bad; fats are an essential part of a healthy diet. The goal is to eat a moderate amount of healthy or unsaturated fatty acids, especially omega-3s, and avoid saturated and trans fat.

What You Should Eat

Understanding these basic concepts, you can now see why you would want to focus on eating lean protein, complex carbohydrates, and a limited amount of healthy fats, while trying to avoid unhealthy fats, sodium, and simple sugars. To do this, your diet should consist primarily of whole grains, fruits and vegetables, and lean protein and fish. In addition, you should try to avoid sweets, fried and fatty foods, and salty foods.

It is easy to think about all the foods that you should avoid, but that is not what will help you be successful in making the life change. Instead, think about all the delicious foods that can be prepared with the types of foods that are optimal for your health and energy. That is what this book will show you. Also think about the balanced weight, increased energy, and decreased risk of the effects and cost of disease on you and your family.

It's Not Just What, It's How Much

What distinguishes the DASH diet from just suggesting eating healthful foods is it offers an optimal amount of the types of foods to eat. Without knowing these amounts, it is easy to eat in excess. If you eat excessive amounts of any food, it will get stored as fat and contribute to obesity, which is unhealthy no matter what food contributed to it. The DASH diet suggests the following amounts:

- Whole Grains: 6–8 daily servings
- Lean Meats or Fish: 6 daily servings or less
- Vegetables: 4–5 daily servings
- Fruits: 4–5 daily servings
- Lean Dairy Products: 2–3 daily servings
- Fats and Oils: 2–3 daily servings or less
- Nuts, Seeds, or Legumes: 4–5 weekly servings
- Sweets and Added Sugars: 5 weekly servings or less

These servings vary based on your caloric needs, but the proportions should stay relatively the same. For example, if you are very active and burn about 3,000 calories per day, you may want to increase whole grains to 9–12 servings, fruits and vegetables to 6–8 servings each, and so on. Similarly, if you are highly inactive, you may want to reduce these amounts somewhat. However, in general, rather than reducing your intake you should—if possible—increase your activity and how many calories you use, as that has many other health benefits.

Putting It All Together

Whole grains, lean meats and fish, and fruits and vegetables are actively encouraged, while fats and sweets are limited. Throughout this book you will be given many examples of foods that fall into the categories of foods that are actively encouraged.

Lean dairy products are also encouraged. This is to ensure you receive an adequate amount of calcium. Of course, some people cannot consume dairy products for various reasons, such as lactose intolerance. In situations where you must avoid a certain food, you just need to understand what beneficial nutrients the food contains and how you can compensate for avoiding it. In the case of lean dairy products, since they supply protein and calcium, it is probably worth increasing lean meat intake slightly and taking a calcium supplement. To best understand what an individual food has that you may be lacking, you can start by reading the nutrition label. Here is an overall summary of the essential ingredients in the types of foods that are recommended:

- Whole Grains—Energy (carbohydrates) and fiber
- Fruits and Vegetables—Potassium, magnesium, and fiber
- Lean Dairy Products—Protein and calcium
- Lean Meats and Fish—Protein and essential fatty acids
- Nuts—Energy (carbohydrates and essential fatty acids), magnesium, potassium, and fiber

In addition to being a source of complex carbohydrates and a low amount of healthy fats, fruits and vegetables are a rich source of vitamins and minerals. By eating more servings of fruits and vegetables, you ensure you get essential amounts of potassium and magnesium. Fruits and vegetables, like whole grains and nuts, also give more fiber. Fiber is a type of carbohydrate that is linked in a way that cannot be absorbed into your bloodstream. Therefore, rather than causing the sugar spike, it attracts fluids into your gut through an osmosis-type effect that adds bulk to your stool and maintains colon health. Since fiber is not absorbed, it can also reduce the absorption of cholesterol and improve your overall cholesterol profile.

FACT

The most important aspect of the DASH diet is eating more of certain types of foods and decreasing certain types of others. Following these basic principles will have a major impact on your health!

What Not to Eat

Most of the foods that are recommended have a very limited amount of sodium, and so should decrease your salt intake. That decrease in salt is one of the biggest benefits of the DASH diet because as discussed, decreasing sodium can directly reduce blood pressure. To be sure that you are limiting your sodium intake, you can look at nutrition labels. In general, it is a good idea to start looking at nutrition labels more, as you will become better acquainted with the various ingredients in the food you eat, which is a huge step to informing and empowering yourself to take control of your health.

Salt

With sodium, the DASH diet actually has two different types of recommendations. The regular DASH diet suggests limiting sodium intake to 2,300 mg daily. If you eat the foods suggested in the DASH diet, you should be able to meet this goal without too much difficulty, but to be sure you can simply add up the sodium content of the various foods you eat to determine your daily total.

ALERT

Not only is too much salt, alcohol, simple sugars, or fat deleterious to your health, but so is too much of nearly any type of food. Excess carbohydrates and good fat create an abundance of calories that are converted to belly fat, which is unhealthy no matter what created it.

The alternative suggestion is for people at especially high risk, including middle-aged to elderly adults, African Americans, and those who already have high blood pressure. For these higher-risk groups, the recommended sodium intake is not to exceed 1,500 mg daily. This is a harder goal to meet without actively paying attention to sodium content, so if you do decide to follow this lower-sodium plan, it is especially important to pay attention to the total sodium on nutrition labels. In addition, if you fall into one of these categories and wish to try to follow the lower-sodium version of the plan, please make sure to talk to your doctor to ensure that such a plan is truly appropriate for you.

Alcohol

Another recommendation of the DASH diet is to limit alcohol intake. Alcohol is known to increase blood pressure and can worsen health. Some studies show a glass of wine daily can improve your cholesterol profile, but this limited benefit may be outweighed by the known harm. The official recommendation of the DASH diet is two or less drinks daily in men and one or less daily in women. Ultimately, though, like sweets and fatty foods, the less alcohol you drink the healthier you will likely be.

Summary

Overall, the DASH diet is not intended to be a temporary change, but rather a sustainable lifestyle. Through the DASH diet, you can reduce your risk of many devastating diseases while achieving an ideal weight and giving yourself more energy. More benefits of the DASH diet are being discovered every day, and it's generally considered by physicians and health institutes as the healthiest diet plan in existence. You have completed the vital task of learning about the DASH diet, and the rest of this book will guide you with delicious recipes to help implement it. You do not need to strictly follow the DASH diet from the first day, as the DASH diet allows gradual change, and forgiveness of imperfection. The DASH diet is a journey, so congratulations on completing the first step.

CHAPTER 2

Appetizers and Snacks

Coconut-Crusted Chicken with Spicy-Sweet Dipping Sauce

Deliciously crisp breading gives way to moist and tender chicken in this healthier alternative to coconut shrimp. A tasty vegan version can be made using tempeh and egg replacement powder.

INGREDIENTS | SERVES 6

4 boneless, skinless chicken thighs (or 8 ounces tempeh)
¼ cup unsweetened coconut
¼ cup salt-free bread crumbs
1 teaspoon garlic powder
¼ teaspoon freshly ground black pepper
1 egg white (or egg replacement powder)
2 tablespoons orange marmalade
1½ teaspoons unflavored rice vinegar
¼ teaspoon dried red pepper flakes

1. Preheat oven to 425°F. Spray a baking sheet lightly with oil and set aside.

2. Wash the chicken and pat dry. Cut the chicken (or tempeh) into 20 bite-sized pieces.

3. Measure the coconut, bread crumbs, garlic powder, and black pepper into a small mixing bowl and whisk well to combine.

4. Place the egg white into a shallow bowl and beat well. (Or prepare egg replacement powder as directed.)

5. Dip each piece of chicken (or tempeh) into the egg, then coat with bread crumbs. Place on prepared baking sheet. Place baking sheet on middle rack in oven and bake 10 minutes.

6. Flip chicken (or tempeh) and return to oven for another 10 minutes (only 5 minutes for the tempeh).

7. While chicken (or tempeh) is baking, measure the marmalade, vinegar, and red pepper flakes into a small bowl and stir well to combine.

8. Remove baking sheet from oven and transfer chicken (or tempeh) to a platter, along with the dipping sauce. Serve immediately.

PER SERVING | Calories: 105 | Fat: 4 g | Protein: 7 g | Sodium: 39 mg | Fiber: 1 g | Carbohydrates: 10 g | Sugar: 5 g

Vegetable Sushi

Although it looks complicated, sushi is simple and inexpensive to make, requiring nothing more than the ingredients, a flexible bamboo sushi mat, and a sharp knife. Dry sheets of nori seaweed are sold in the Asian aisle of most supermarkets. Sushi rice, sometimes called sticky rice, should also be there. If you don't see it, ask.

INGREDIENTS | SERVES 6

2 cups sushi rice

3 cups water

1 medium carrot

1 medium cucumber

2 tablespoons unflavored rice vinegar

5 sheets unflavored nori

Sushi Tip

When making sushi, position a bowl of water nearby on the counter. Dip your sticky fingers into the water to make rice arrangement easier, and use it to rinse your knife for clean and pressure-free slicing.

1. Place the rice and water into a saucepan and bring to a boil over high heat. Once boiling, reduce heat to low and simmer, covered, 20 minutes.

2. While rice is cooking, peel the carrot and cucumber. Remove the cucumber seeds by halving lengthwise, then gently scraping seeds out with a spoon. Slice the carrot and cucumber into thin matchsticks or strips and set aside.

3. When the rice is done, remove from heat. Add the rice vinegar and mix well.

4. Take out a sheet of nori. One side should be shinier than the other; place the shiny side down on the bamboo mat. Spread a thin layer of rice (roughly ¼-inch thick) over top, leaving a 1-inch bare lip near you and about 2 inches bare on the far edge.

5. Place a strip of carrots and/or cucumber on top of the rice, about 2 to 3 inches from the bare edge closest to you. Lightly wet the bare edges, then carefully roll the nori away from you, pressing firmly to seal. Continue rolling to the far edge, then roll back and forth to seal completely.

6. Using a very sharp knife, slice the roll into 7 equal segments, dipping the knife into water and cleaning the blade off between cuts to prevent sticking.

7. Serve sushi immediately or cover and refrigerate until serving.

PER SERVING | Calories: 73 | Fat: 0 g | Protein: 2 g | Sodium: 15 mg | Fiber: 1 g | Carbohydrates: 15 g | Sugar: 2 g

Zucchini Sticks

Modeled after fried mozzarella, these yummy zucchini sticks are crisp and golden on the outside and tender inside.

INGREDIENTS | SERVES 6

2 small–medium zucchini

1 egg white

1 tablespoon water

3 tablespoons salt-free bread crumbs

1 tablespoon grated Parmesan cheese

1 teaspoon dried Italian seasoning

½ teaspoon garlic powder

½ teaspoon onion powder

¼ teaspoon freshly ground black pepper

⅛ teaspoon ground sweet paprika

½ cup no-salt-added pasta sauce

For the Love of Zucchini

Easy to grow and notoriously prodigious, zucchini is a garden favorite. When planting, leave plenty of space for the specimens to spread. The leaves of zucchini plants and the vegetables themselves can grow to massive proportions. Zucchini are best harvested when young and tender; older specimens can become tough and unappealing. The flowers of the plant are also edible. Many farmers' markets now offer zucchini blossoms for sale; keep an eye out when shopping.

1. Preheat oven to 450°F. Spray a baking sheet lightly with oil and set aside.

2. Trim ends off the zucchinis, then cut in half. Quarter each of these halves, to make 16 (roughly) equal wedges.

3. Beat the egg white and water in a small shallow bowl. Set aside.

4. Place the bread crumbs, cheese, and seasonings into a small mixing bowl and whisk well to combine.

5. Dip each piece of zucchini in egg, then roll in bread crumbs. Place on baking sheet. Place baking sheet on middle rack in oven and bake for 15 minutes.

6. While zucchini is baking, gently warm pasta sauce on stovetop or in microwave. Pour into a small bowl and set aside.

7. Remove zucchini sticks from oven and serve immediately with warm sauce.

PER SERVING | Calories: 39 | Fat: 1 g | Protein: 2 g | Sodium: 28 mg | Fiber: 1 g | Carbohydrates: 6 g | Sugar: 2 g

Mushroom, Swiss, and Jalapeño Quesadillas

*Two tortillas lightly grilled, with a spicy, cheesy, savory filling. What could be better?
Perfect as appetizers or a light meal, these quesadillas leave processed fast food in the dust,
where it should be. If spicy food's not your thing, simply omit the jalapeño.*

INGREDIENTS | SERVES 8

1 teaspoon olive oil

1 pound fresh mushrooms, sliced

1 medium onion, diced

3 cloves garlic, minced

Freshly ground black pepper, to taste

1 (12-ounce) package Garden City Brand All Natural Lavash Roll-Ups or equivalent

1 cup shredded Swiss cheese

1 jalapeño pepper, sliced

2 tablespoons chopped fresh cilantro

¼ cup nonfat sour cream

Garden City All Natural Lavash Roll-Ups

Sold at Whole Foods markets, these round tortilla-like wraps are a perfect choice for low-sodium dieters. They're sold in white or whole-wheat versions, and contain a mere 20 mg sodium per serving. Garden City lavash are stocked in the bakery department near the bread, typically on an inconspicuous lower shelf. If you don't see them, ask.

1. Heat oil in a skillet over medium heat. Add mushrooms, onion, and garlic and cook, stirring, until brown and tender, about 10 minutes. Season with freshly ground pepper to taste.

2. Heat a large nonstick skillet or griddle over medium-low heat. Place a single lavash on surface, flipping once or twice to warm, then sprinkle ½ cup cheese, half of the jalapeño slices, and half the cilantro evenly over top.

3. Wait a few minutes for cheese to melt, then spread with half of the mushroom mixture. Sandwich with a second lavash, then carefully flip the entire quesadilla over to toast on the second side.

4. Once second side has crisped a bit, remove from griddle and place on a clean, flat surface. Using a pizza cutter or sharp knife, slice quesadilla into quarters, then cut each quarter in half, leaving 8 pieces.

5. Repeat process with remaining ingredients.

6. Serve hot, garnished with nonfat sour cream.

PER SERVING | Calories: 192 | Fat: 6 g | Protein: 10 g | Sodium: 103 mg | Fiber: 2 g | Carbohydrates: 28 g | Sugar: 2 g

Heavenly Deviled Eggs

Creamy, tart, and addictive. To easily remove the shells from the cooked eggs, crack against a hard surface, then hold under cool running water. The peels should slide right off.

INGREDIENTS | SERVES 6

6 eggs

1 tablespoon nonfat sour cream

1 tablespoon water or low-sodium chicken broth

1 tablespoon finely chopped fresh chives

1 teaspoon no-salt-added prepared mustard

½ teaspoon dried herbes de Provence

Freshly ground black pepper, to taste

Ground sweet paprika, for garnish

Snipping Versus Slicing

When working with fresh herbs such as chives, it's often far easier to snip them into small pieces using a pair of kitchen shears than to slice through them with a knife. A good pair of kitchen scissors can be purchased inexpensively and is worth the small investment for the savings in time alone.

1. Place eggs in a saucepan and add enough water to cover them by a couple inches. Bring to a boil over high heat; lower heat slightly, and boil 12 minutes.

2. Remove pan from heat, place in sink under cold running water, and let sit 1–2 minutes until eggs are cool enough to handle.

3. Peel eggs and slice in half lengthwise. Gently remove yolks and place in a small mixing bowl.

4. To the yolks, add the sour cream, water (or broth), chives, and mustard. Stir well to combine.

5. Crush the herbs in your hand and add to the mixture, along with freshly ground black pepper, to taste. Mix until smooth.

6. Divide the yolk mixture evenly among the egg halves, filling neatly. Sprinkle with ground paprika and serve.

PER SERVING | Calories: 79 | Fat: 5 g | Protein: 6 g | Sodium: 66 mg | Fiber: 0 g | Carbohydrates: 1 g | Sugar: 0 g

Spice-Rubbed Chicken Wings

These flavorful wings are great for casual parties or game day get-togethers.
The spice rub works well on other cuts of chicken, from thighs to drumsticks, even whole birds.
For more heat, add a pinch of ground cayenne pepper to the blend.

INGREDIENTS | SERVES 6

3 pounds chicken wings
2 teaspoons ground cumin
1 teaspoon ground coriander
1 teaspoon dry ground mustard
1 teaspoon garlic powder
1 teaspoon onion powder
½ teaspoon freshly ground black pepper
¼ teaspoon dried red pepper flakes
¼ teaspoon ground sweet paprika

Waste Not, Want Not

Animal bones can't be composted, but they can be used to flavor recipes, especially homemade broth. Place bones and other scraps in a stockpot, add water, and bring to a boil over high heat. Once boiling, reduce heat to low, cover, and simmer an hour or more. When it comes to vegetable trimmings, do the same. Peels, leaves, and stems may be unappealing to eat, but add a lot of flavor to stock. Save discarded scraps in plastic bags, seal, and freeze for later use.

1. Wash and pat chicken wings dry. Sever wing tips at joint and save for later use.

2. Place seasonings into a mixing bowl and whisk well to combine.

3. Rub wings all over with spice mixture. Place wings into mixing bowl, cover, and refrigerate several hours or overnight.

4. When ready to cook, heat grill to medium heat or preheat oven to 450°F.

5. If grilling, place wings on grates and grill 20 minutes, flipping frequently to prevent burning. Keep wings away from direct flame. The wings are done when an internal temperature of 180°F is reached.

6. If roasting in oven, place wings on a lightly oiled baking sheet. Place sheet on middle rack in oven and bake 15 minutes. Flip the wings, return to oven, and bake another 15 minutes.

7. Serve immediately.

PER SERVING | Calories: 464 | Fat: 18 g | Protein: 64 g | Sodium: 185 mg | Fiber: 0 g | Carbohydrates: 1 g | Sugar: 0 g

Savory Stuffed Mushrooms

A lovely appetizer or light nosh, these salt-free stuffed mushrooms have a crisp and tasty breading that's so good, they'll be gone before you know it. Great with white button or baby bella mushrooms.

INGREDIENTS | SERVES 6

16 ounces fresh mushrooms
2 tablespoons olive oil
½ cup salt-free bread crumbs
1 egg white
½ cup shredded Swiss cheese
4 cloves garlic
1 teaspoon dried Italian seasoning
½ teaspoon freshly ground black pepper

1. Preheat oven to 400°F. Spray a baking sheet lightly with oil and set aside.

2. Clean the mushrooms and gently remove stems, taking care to leave the caps intact. Set caps aside.

3. Place the mushroom stems in a food processor and add the remaining ingredients. Pulse several times to finely chop and combine the mixture.

4. Stuff each mushroom cap with the mixture, then place on the prepared baking sheet. Place pan on middle rack in oven and bake 15 minutes. Remove from oven.

5. Mushrooms can be served warm or at room temperature.

PER SERVING | Calories: 124 | Fat: 7 g | Protein: 5 g | Sodium: 30 mg | Fiber: 1 g | Carbohydrates: 10 g | Sugar: 1 g

Baked Tofu with Tangy Dipping Sauce

Anything but bland, these breaded, oven-fried cutlets will make a tofu lover out of you! Paired with a sweet, slightly spicy sauce, they're absolutely delicious. Double the quantity of tofu for larger parties.

INGREDIENTS | SERVES 8

1 pound extra-firm tofu, drained

1 egg white

1 tablespoon water

½ cup salt-free bread crumbs

1 tablespoon dried parsley

1 teaspoon dried Italian seasoning

1 teaspoon ground sweet paprika

1 teaspoon onion powder

½ teaspoon garlic powder

½ teaspoon freshly ground black pepper

1 (8-ounce) can no-salt-added tomato sauce

1 tablespoon apple cider vinegar

1 tablespoon molasses

1 tablespoon honey

1 tablespoon dry ground mustard

½ teaspoon ground cumin

Pinch ground cayenne pepper

What Is Tofu?

Tofu is made from soy beans in a process not unlike the making of cheese. Bean curds are separated from liquid and pressed into blocks. Tofu is sold in two main types. The first type, what many consider "regular" tofu, is sold in blocks submerged in liquid. It comes in silken, firm, and extra-firm varieties and must be kept refrigerated. The second type of tofu, which comes in shelf-stable packaging and does not need to be refrigerated, is silken style. It comes in varying levels of firmness, from silken to extra firm; all have a soft, smooth feel.

1. Preheat oven to 425°F. Spray a baking sheet lightly with oil and set aside.

2. Gently press the drained tofu between paper towels to release excess liquid. Slice tofu in half lengthwise, then slice each half into 8 equal pieces.

3. Beat the egg white and water in a shallow bowl until slightly foamy.

4. Place the bread crumbs into a bowl, add the seasonings (parsley through black pepper), and whisk well to combine.

5. Dip each piece of tofu in egg white, then gently press in the bread crumbs to coat. Place coated tofu cutlets on prepared baking sheet.

6. Place baking sheet on middle rack in oven and bake 10 minutes. Remove from oven, gently flip, and return to oven to bake another 10 minutes.

7. While tofu is baking, combine tomato sauce and remaining ingredients in a saucepan. Heat over medium-low heat, stirring frequently. Once mixture begins to bubble, remove from heat and pour into a small serving bowl.

8. Remove tofu from oven and serve immediately with tangy dipping sauce.

PER SERVING | Calories: 121 | Fat: 3 g | Protein: 8 g | Sodium: 15 mg | Fiber: 2 g | Carbohydrates: 15 g | Sugar: 6 g

Sweet and Spicy Salt-Free Pickles

With a brine this sassy, you won't notice the lack of salt, and it's great for pickling other vegetables, too. The flavor increases the longer the cucumbers marinate, so these are best made at least a day before serving.

INGREDIENTS | YIELDS 10 CUPS

3 large cucumbers
1 medium onion, thinly sliced
6 cloves garlic, minced
4 cups white vinegar
2 cups sugar
1 tablespoon mustard seed
3 bay leaves
1 teaspoon dried red pepper flakes
½ teaspoon whole peppercorns

1. Wash the cucumbers and slice into thin rounds. Peel and trim the onion, and slice thinly.

2. Place the sliced cucumber, onion, and minced garlic into a large lidded jar or other airtight container.

3. Add the remaining ingredients to a saucepan and stir well to combine. Bring to a boil over medium heat, stirring occasionally. Once boiling, remove from heat and pour over mixture in jar.

4. Screw on lid and let sit until cool.

5. Once cool, store in refrigerator. Pickles will keep for several weeks in refrigerator.

PER SERVING (¼ CUP) | Calories: 23 | Fat: 0 g | Protein: 0 g | Sodium: 2 mg | Fiber: 0 g | Carbohydrates: 4 g | Sugar: 3 g

Crunchy Coated Nuts

Slightly sweet, with a spicy kick from the cayenne, these crunchy nuts are the life of any party. If you prefer less heat, reduce the amount of cayenne pepper. Recipe adapted from Food Network Kitchens Favorite Recipes.

INGREDIENTS | SERVES 8

1 egg white
3 tablespoons brown sugar
2 teaspoons dried oregano
¾ teaspoon ground coriander
½ teaspoon ground cumin
¼ teaspoon ground cayenne pepper
Small pinch ground cloves
2 cups unsalted mixed nuts

Healthy Homemade Gifts

The most thoughtful gifts are often those you make yourself. Packaging unsalted nuts and other salt-free snacks in tins or glass containers is a tasty way of showing you care. At holiday time, there's nothing sweeter than sharing a tray of healthy, home-baked sweets. And remember, salt-free seasonings and condiments are practical as well as delicious. Placed in a pretty jar or squeeze bottle, they're a gift that keeps on giving.

1. Preheat oven to 300°F. Line a sided baking sheet with parchment or aluminum foil.

2. Place the egg white and seasonings in a small mixing bowl and whisk until well combined.

3. Add the mixed nuts and toss until evenly coated.

4. Arrange the nuts in a single layer on the baking sheet.

5. Place the baking sheet on the middle rack in the oven and bake 30 minutes, removing the pan halfway through baking time, stirring well, and returning to oven.

6. Remove baking sheet from oven and set on wire rack to cool. Nuts will crisp as they dry and cool, so let them cool fully before removing from the sheet. Store in an airtight container for up to 5 days.

PER SERVING | Calories: 226 | Fat: 17 g | Protein: 6 g | Sodium: 13 mg | Fiber: 3 g | Carbohydrates: 14 g | Sugar: 5 g

Cheesy Seasoned Popcorn

This seasoned popcorn will satisfy salty snack cravings anytime.
Experiment with different herbs or try a sugar-and-spice blend, as suggested below.

INGREDIENTS | YIELDS 10 CUPS

2 tablespoons nutritional yeast flakes
1½ teaspoons dried dill
1 teaspoon dried parsley
¾ teaspoon garlic powder
¾ teaspoon onion powder
½ teaspoon ground sweet paprika
¼ teaspoon dried thyme
¼ teaspoon freshly ground black pepper
½ cup popcorn kernels
2 teaspoons olive oil

1. Measure the nutritional yeast, dill, parsley, garlic powder, onion powder, paprika, thyme, and black pepper into a small bowl and stir well to combine. Set aside.

2. Place popcorn kernels into an air popper. Place a stockpot beneath the popcorn dispenser, turn appliance on, and wait until kernels have popped. Turn off popper and set aside.

3. Drizzle the oil over the popcorn and toss well to coat. Once popcorn is thoroughly coated with oil, sprinkle with the seasoning mixture and stir vigorously for several minutes until completely coated.

4. Serve immediately or store in an airtight container until serving.

PER SERVING (1 CUP) | Calories: 55 | Fat: 1 g | Protein: 2 g | Sodium: 2 mg | Fiber: 2 g | Carbohydrates: 8 g | Sugar: <1 g

Salt-Free Tos

Lip-smacking, finger-licking good, and completely salt free! These homemade seasoned tortilla chips are just like your old favorites, but better. Benson's Salt-Free Seasonings are sold online at www.bensonsgourmetseasonings.com.

INGREDIENTS | SERVES 6

3 tablespoons nutritional yeast flakes (e.g., Red Star)

1½ tablespoons Benson's Table Tasty

1 tablespoon Benson's Bravado

10 small (5-inch) corn tortillas

1 cup canola oil (for frying)

Chef's Note

Although fried, only a fraction of the oil in this recipe is absorbed into the chips, the rest drains off onto paper towels. Nutritional yeast, such as Red Star, is sold at health food stores and some supermarkets, often with the baking products, seasonings, or bulk foods. Its salty, cheese-like taste adds a tremendous low-sodium boost to many foods.

1. Measure the nutritional yeast and seasonings into a small paper bag. Close securely and shake well to combine. Set aside.

2. Stack the tortillas, 3 or 4 at a time, and cut into 6 equal-sized wedges using a pizza cutter or sharp knife. Repeat process with all of the tortillas, until you have a total of 60 wedges or chips.

3. Place paper towels on a baking sheet and set aside.

4. Heat the oil in a skillet over medium. Once oil is hot, add several wedges to the pan, being careful not to overcrowd. The chips cook quickly and have a tendency to stick together. Cook until crisp and golden, roughly 30 seconds, then remove from pan and place on paper towels to drain. If chips begin to brown too quickly, lower heat immediately.

5. When chips have drained, place in the paper bag with the seasonings. Close securely and shake well to coat. Remove chips from bag and place on a wire rack to cool.

6. Repeat process until all chips are cooked and seasoned.

7. Serve immediately or store in an airtight container until serving.

PER SERVING | Calories: 130 | Fat: 5 g | Protein: 1 g | Sodium: 8 mg | Fiber: 2 g | Carbohydrates: 17 g | Sugar: 2 g

Salt-Free Trail Mix

A chewy and filling combination of dried fruit and unsalted nuts makes low-sodium snacking a breeze. Vary dried fruit according to taste; feel free to add chocolate or carob chips to the mix, too.

INGREDIENTS | YIELDS 16 SERVINGS

½ cup seedless raisins
½ cup dried cranberries
½ cup dried apricots
½ cup dried pitted dates
½ cup unsalted sunflower seeds
½ cup unsalted cashews
½ cup unsalted peanuts
½ cup unsalted almonds

1. Place all the ingredients into a mixing bowl and stir well to combine.

2. Store in an airtight container until serving.

PER SERVING | Calories: 146 | Fat: 8 g | Protein: 3 g | Sodium: 2 mg | Fiber: 2 g | Carbohydrates: 17 g | Sugar: 11 g

Seasoned Sesame Kale Chips

Light as air, crisp, and addictive, these chips get their salty taste from low-sodium kale seasoning. Another salt-free seasoning may be substituted if preferred.

INGREDIENTS | SERVES 4

1 bunch fresh kale

2½ teaspoons Bragg Organic Sea Kelp Delight Seasoning

2 teaspoons toasted sesame seeds

What Is Kelp?

Kelp is a type of harvested seaweed. It's naturally low in sodium with a pronounced salty taste, making it an excellent salt substitute. Kelp is low in fat and calories, aids metabolism through its high concentration of iodine, and is a great source of vitamin K and folate. Kelp is sold in dried form, either alone or as part of a seasoning blend. Maine Coast Sea Vegetables Organic Kelp Granules and Bragg Organic Sea Kelp Delight Seasoning are two such products; both are sold in select stores and online.

1. Preheat oven to 325°F. Lightly spray a baking sheet with oil and set aside.

2. Wash kale and pat dry. Remove leaves from the tough stalks, cut or tear into pieces, and arrange in a single layer on the baking sheet.

3. Spray lightly with oil and sprinkle with seasoning and sesame seeds.

4. Place baking sheet on middle rack in oven and bake 12 minutes. Remove from oven and transfer chips to a sheet of waxed paper or foil to cool. Repeat process with remaining ingredients.

5. Store in an airtight container.

PER SERVING | Calories: 41 | Fat: 1 g | Protein: 2 g | Sodium: 77 mg | Fiber: 2 g | Carbohydrates: 7 g | Sugar: 0 g

Sweet Potato Crisps

Love store-bought sweet potato chips? This homemade version is so good you may never buy them again. Adapted from Chow.com.

INGREDIENTS | SERVES 2

1 medium sweet potato, scrubbed well
2 teaspoons olive oil
½ teaspoon ground sweet paprika

1. Position 2 oven racks in the middle of the oven. Preheat oven to 350°F. Get out 2 baking sheets and set aside.

2. Slice the sweet potato into paper-thin rounds using a mandolin or very sharp knife.

3. Place slices into a mixing bowl, add the oil and paprika, and toss well to coat. Arrange the slices in a single layer on the baking sheets. Do not overlap.

4. Place the baking sheets on the middle 2 racks in the oven and bake 8 minutes. Switch the baking sheet positions and bake another 7–8 minutes, until the edges of the slices begin to curl and the centers are golden brown and dry to the touch.

5. Remove baking sheets from the oven and place on wire racks. Cool for a few minutes before transferring to a bowl. Serve immediately or store in an airtight container for up to 3 days.

PER SERVING | Calories: 93 | Fat: 4 g | Protein: 1 g | Sodium: 21 mg | Fiber: 2 g | Carbohydrates: 12 g | Sugar: 4 g

Chewy Granola Bars

These soft and chewy granola bars make a healthy, fat-free change from their commercial counterparts. Perfect for a quick energy boost or a guilt-free go-to snack anytime. Adapted from WomenHeart's All Heart Family Cookbook.

INGREDIENTS | YIELDS 20 BARS

3 cups quick oats

1 cup white whole-wheat flour

2 teaspoons sodium-free baking soda

1 teaspoon ground cinnamon

¼ teaspoon ground nutmeg

1½ cups unsweetened applesauce

¾ cup brown sugar

2 teaspoons pure vanilla extract

⅔ cup raisins or dried cranberries

Differences in Oats

Oats come in three main types. Quick or instant oats have been precooked and dried. They have the fastest cooking time and are great for making oatmeal or adding to baked goods. Old-fashioned rolled oats have been put through a steaming process to speed cooking. They're considered all-purpose and work well in most recipes. Steel-cut oats, sometimes labeled Scotch or Irish, are cut, not rolled. They have a chewy texture that's good for oatmeal and other recipes, but because of their longer cooking time, aren't ideal for everything.

1. Preheat oven to 350°F. Spray two 8-inch square baking pans lightly with oil and set aside.

2. Place the oats, flour, baking soda, cinnamon, and nutmeg into a mixing bowl and whisk well to combine.

3. Add the applesauce, brown sugar, and vanilla and mix well. Stir in the dried fruit. Divide the mixture evenly between the 2 prepared pans and smooth down. Place pans on the middle rack in oven and bake 20 minutes.

4. Remove pans from oven and place on wire rack to cool briefly. Cut each pan into 10 equal-size bars. Carefully remove bars from pans and place on wire rack to cool. Serve immediately, store in an airtight container, or wrap individually and freeze.

PER SERVING | Calories: 122 | Fat: 1 g | Protein: 2 g | Sodium: 4 mg | Fiber: 2 g | Carbohydrates: 27 g | Sugar: 13 g

Fresh Fruit with Almond Banana Butter

Serve with ripe cantaloupe, pineapple, grapes, apples, pears, and strawberries for a delectable party tray. Almond banana butter also makes a healthy low-sodium sandwich spread.

INGREDIENTS | SERVES 8

Assorted fresh fruit

½ cup unsalted almonds

1 ripe banana

1 tablespoon honey (optional)

Almond Facts

The almond tree is related to the peach and cherry, and produces similar blossoms and stone-like fruit. In the case of almonds, however, the fruit is actually the inner pit, encased in a hard outer shell. The nuts can be eaten whole, ground into a flour, or consumed as a paste similar to peanut butter. Almonds are high in monounsaturated fats and vitamin E, and have been shown to help reduce cholesterol and the risk of heart disease.

1. Wash fruit and cut into chunks or thread onto skewers. Arrange on a platter and set aside.

2. Place the almonds into a blender or food processor and purée.

3. Add the banana and honey (if using) and purée until smooth. Transfer the mixture to a small serving bowl and place beside fruit.

4. Serve immediately.

PER SERVING (ALMOND BANANA BUTTER ONLY) | Calories: 72 | Fat: 4 g | Protein: 2 g | Sodium: <1 mg | Fiber: 1 g | Carbohydrates: 7 g | Sugar: 4 g

CHAPTER 3

Biscuits, Muffins, Scones, and Quick Breads

Baking Powder Biscuits

These light and flaky biscuits are table ready in 15 minutes, making them a great choice for any meal. Substitute unsalted butter for the shortening if you prefer.

INGREDIENTS | YIELDS 1 DOZEN

1 cup unbleached all-purpose flour

1 cup white whole-wheat flour

1 tablespoon sugar

4 teaspoons sodium-free baking powder

4 tablespoons nonhydrogenated vegetable shortening (e.g., Spectrum Naturals)

1 egg white

⅔ cup low-fat milk

Nonhydrogenated Vegetable Shortening

Traditional vegetable shortening is made by adding hydrogen to liquid oil, rendering it solid. This chemical process produces trans fats, fatty acids linked to coronary heart disease and high cholesterol. Nonhydrogenated vegetable shortening is made naturally from pressed oils that are solid at room temperature. It's trans fat free as well as cholesterol free, making it a good alternative to butter when baking. Spectrum Naturals Organic All Vegetable Shortening is sold at Whole Foods markets and online.

1. Preheat oven to 450°F. Take out a baking sheet and set aside.

2. Place the flour, sugar, and baking powder into a mixing bowl and whisk well to combine.

3. Cut the shortening into the mixture using your fingers, and work until it resembles coarse crumbs. Add the egg white and milk and stir to combine.

4. Turn the dough out onto a lightly floured surface and knead 1 minute. Roll dough to (roughly) ¾-inch thickness and cut into 12 (2-inch) rounds.

5. Place rounds on the baking sheet. Place baking sheet on middle rack in oven and bake 10 minutes.

6. Remove baking sheet and place biscuits on a wire rack to cool.

PER SERVING | Calories: 118 | Fat: 4 g | Protein: 3 g | Sodium: 13 mg | Fiber: 1 g | Carbohydrates: 16 g | Sugar: <1 g

Sweet Potato Biscuits

Worry-free biscuits with a sweet potato twist, these are easy to make and even easier to eat. Adapted from Food Network Kitchens Favorite Recipes.

INGREDIENTS | YIELDS 8

1 medium sweet potato, peeled and cut into small chunks

1 cup unbleached all-purpose flour

½ cup white whole-wheat flour

1 tablespoon sodium-free baking powder

1 tablespoon brown sugar

½ teaspoon ground cinnamon

⅛ teaspoon ground allspice

4 tablespoons unsalted butter

½ cup low fat milk

1. Preheat oven to 425°F. Take out a baking sheet, line it with 2 sheets of parchment, and set aside.

2. Place sweet potato in a small saucepan, cover with water, and bring to a boil. Lower heat and boil until sweet potato is soft, roughly 15 minutes.

3. Remove pan from heat, drain, then mash the sweet potato well. Measure out ¾ cup and set aside. Reserve any remaining purée for another use.

4. Place the flour, baking powder, brown sugar, cinnamon, and allspice into a mixing bowl and whisk together. Add the butter and cut into the dry mixture using your fingertips. Process the dough until the butter is broken down to roughly pea-sized pieces.

5. Add the mashed sweet potato and milk and mix to form a moist dough.

6. Turn out on a lightly floured surface and pat dough into a rectangle about ½-inch thick. Fold dough into thirds, as if folding a business letter, then pat lightly into a (roughly) 8" × 5" rectangle about ¾-inch thick.

7. Using a 2-inch round biscuit cutter, cut out 6 biscuits, then gently transfer to baking sheet. Pat the dough scraps together to form another small rectangle, then cut out 2 more biscuits. Transfer to baking sheet.

8. Place baking sheet on middle rack in oven and bake 12 minutes, until lightly browned. Remove from oven and place on a wire rack to cool.

PER SERVING | Calories: 160 | Fat: 6 g | Protein: 3 g | Sodium: 15 mg | Fiber: 2 g | Carbohydrates: 23 g | Sugar: 3 g

Whole-Grain Crackers with Rosemary, Garlic, and Parmesan

These crisp salt-free crackers make super snacks. Partner with soup, sliced Swiss cheese, and crunchy grapes for a wonderful light meal.

INGREDIENTS | YIELDS 6½ DOZEN

1⅔ cups white whole-wheat flour

½ teaspoon sodium-free baking powder

1 tablespoon all-purpose salt-free seasoning

1 teaspoon ground rosemary

1 teaspoon garlic powder

½ cup low-fat milk

¼ cup grated Parmesan cheese

3 tablespoons olive oil

1 egg white

1–2 tablespoons water, if needed

Parmesan Cheese

Parmesan cheese can add a lot of flavor, but it can also add unwanted fat and sodium. When selecting a cheese, check nutrition facts carefully. BelGioioso Grated Parmesan is one of the lowest in both fat and sodium, containing only 1 g fat per tablespoon and a mere 45 mg sodium. Bel-Gioioso is sold in many supermarkets and specialty cheese shops.

1. Preheat oven to 400°F. Spray a baking sheet lightly with oil and set aside.

2. Place the flour, baking powder, and seasonings into a mixing bowl and whisk well to combine.

3. Add the milk, cheese, oil, and egg white and stir to make a stiff dough. Add 1–2 tablespoons of water if the dough is still a little too dry.

4. Turn the dough out onto a lightly floured surface and knead several minutes, until dough is smooth and intact. Roll out to roughly ⅛-inch thickness, no thinner or the crackers will burn. Cut into 1½-inch squares and transfer to the prepared baking sheet.

5. Place baking sheet on middle rack in oven and bake 10 minutes. Remove from oven and place crackers on wire rack to cool. Once cool, store in an airtight container.

PER SERVING (6 CRACKERS) | Calories: 95 | Fat: 4 g | Protein: 3 g | Sodium: 38 mg | Fiber: 2 g | Carbohydrates: 12 g | Sugar: 1 g

Homemade Soft Pretzels

Delicious, hot-from-the-oven soft pretzels are easier to make than you'd think.
After baking, spray lightly with oil and sprinkle with choice of seasoning, enjoy plain,
or serve with salt-free mustard.

INGREDIENTS | YIELDS 10

4½ teaspoons dry active yeast

1½ cups warm water

2 tablespoons honey

3 cups unbleached all-purpose flour

1 cup white whole-wheat flour

1 egg, beaten (for brushing)

1. Preheat oven to 425°F. Take out a large baking sheet and set aside.

2. Place the yeast into a large mixing bowl. Add water, honey, and flours and stir to combine. Turn dough out onto a lightly floured surface and knead 5 minutes.

3. Divide dough into 10 equal pieces. Roll each piece into a long snake-like tube, then twist to form a pretzel. Place pretzels onto the baking sheet and brush lightly with the beaten egg.

4. Place baking sheet on middle rack in oven and bake 15 minutes, until golden brown. Remove from oven and place pretzels on a wire rack to cool.

PER SERVING | Calories: 200 | Fat: 1 g | Protein: 6 g | Sodium: 8 mg | Fiber: 3 g | Carbohydrates: 41 g | Sugar: 4 g

Soft and Crusty No-Rise Bread

Low-sodium dieters despair no more! This quick and easy recipe yields a fabulous loaf of bread, dinner, or sandwich rolls in 30 minutes or less. Brushing the bread with beaten egg before baking gives it a gloriously glossy, golden crust.

INGREDIENTS | YIELDS 1 LOAF, 8 SANDWICH ROLLS, OR 12 DINNER ROLLS

1 tablespoon dry active yeast

2 teaspoons olive oil

1 tablespoon sugar

1 teaspoon all-purpose salt-free seasoning

1¼ cups warm water

1¼ cups unbleached all-purpose flour

1 cup white whole-wheat flour

1 beaten egg, for brushing

All-Purpose Salt-Free Seasoning

If there's a single seasoning to find on a low-sodium diet, it's this one! All-purpose salt-free seasoning is a unique blend of herbs, spices, dehydrated vegetables, citrus zest, and sometimes nutritional yeast. Its combination of flavors can replace salt at the table and in recipes, with no additional sodium. Some excellent brands are Bensons Table Tasty, Olde Thompson Organic No Salt Seasoning, and Frontier All-Purpose Seasoning Salt-Free Blend. Try as many different blends and brands as possible until you find one or more you truly love.

1. Preheat oven to 425°F. Spray a baking sheet lightly with oil and set aside.

2. Place the yeast, olive oil, sugar, and seasoning into a large mixing bowl and add the water. Gradually add in the flours, stirring well to combine.

3. Once dough comes together, turn out onto a lightly floured surface and knead, adding up to ¼ cup additional flour as necessary. Knead 5 minutes, until dough is smooth and elastic.

4. Shape loaf as desired or cut into 8 or 12 equal portions and roll into buns or rolls. Place on prepared baking sheet and brush lightly with beaten egg.

5. Place pan on middle rack in oven and bake 15 minutes for 12 dinner rolls, 20 minutes for 8 sandwich rolls, or 30 minutes for a single loaf.

6. Remove from oven and serve immediately, or transfer to a wire rack to cool.

PER SERVING (12 SERVINGS) | Calories: 100 | Fat: 1 g | Protein: 3 g | Sodium: 7 mg | Fiber: 1 g | Carbohydrates: 18 g | Sugar: 1 g

Irish Soda Bread

Authentic Irish soda bread seems to be a matter of debate. Many American recipes call for eggs, caraway seeds, and raisins and produce loaves much like tea cake. Other recipes add potato flour or rolled oats, yielding the exact opposite—much heartier loaves without a hint of sweetness. This recipe aims for the latter, producing a heavy, salt-free bread with a good crust, lovely toasted with or without butter.

INGREDIENTS | YIELDS 2 SMALL LOAVES

1¼ cups low-fat milk
4 teaspoons distilled white vinegar
2 cups unbleached all-purpose flour
1 cup white whole-wheat flour
2 teaspoons sodium-free baking soda
3 tablespoons sugar

1. Preheat oven to 400°F. Spray a baking sheet lightly with oil and set aside.

2. Pour the milk into a small bowl or measuring cup, add the vinegar, and set aside 5 minutes.

3. Place the dry ingredients into a large mixing bowl and whisk well to combine.

4. Add the milk and stir, first using a spoon, then your hands. Gather the dough up into a ball, place on a floured surface, and knead very briefly, just to smooth the dough and incorporate ingredients fully.

5. Divide dough into 2 equal portions and shape into small round loaves. Place loaves onto the prepared baking sheet and score an "X" on the top of each using a sharp knife. Gently sift a little flour over top.

6. Place baking sheet on the middle rack in the oven and bake 30 minutes. Remove from oven and place on wire rack to cool. Cool fully before slicing and serving.

PER SERVING (12 SERVINGS) | Calories: 133 | Fat: <1 g | Protein: 4 g | Sodium: 12 mg | Fiber: 2 g | Carbohydrates: 27 g | Sugar: 5 g

Perfect Cornbread

This foolproof cornbread strikes the ideal balance between sweet and savory.
Substitute white whole-wheat flour for all-purpose if desired.

INGREDIENTS | SERVES 16

1 cup cornmeal
¾ cup unbleached all-purpose flour
1 tablespoon sodium-free baking powder
⅓ cup sugar or maple syrup
1 cup low-fat milk
1 egg white
¼ cup canola oil
1 teaspoon pure vanilla extract

1. Preheat oven to 425°F. Grease an 8-inch baking pan and set aside.

2. Place ingredients into a mixing bowl and stir well to combine. Pour batter into prepared pan. Place pan on middle rack in oven and bake for 20 minutes.

3. Remove from oven and place on a wire rack to cool. Cool briefly before cutting into squares and serving.

PER SERVING | Calories: 103 | Fat: 4 g | Protein: 2 g | Sodium: 13 mg | Fiber: 1 g | Carbohydrates: 15 g | Sugar: 5 g

Fabulous Fat-Free Cornbread!

Make an equally delicious fat-free version of this cornbread by substituting ¼ cup unsweetened applesauce for the canola oil and skim milk for the low-fat milk. Add ½ cup frozen corn to the batter for an added treat.

Salt-Free Croutons

Here's a tasty way to use leftover low-sodium bread.
These delicious croutons will dress up any green salad or enhance even the simplest of soups.

INGREDIENTS | YIELDS 4 CUPS

6 cups cubed salt-free bread

2 tablespoons olive oil

1½ tablespoons grated Parmesan cheese

1 teaspoon dried Italian seasoning

1 teaspoon garlic powder

1. Preheat oven to 350°F. Take out a baking sheet and set aside.

2. Place all the ingredients into a mixing bowl and toss well to coat. Spread bread cubes evenly on a baking sheet. Place sheet on middle rack in oven and bake for 10 minutes.

3. Remove from oven and place on wire rack to cool. Store in an airtight container until ready to serve.

PER SERVING (¼ CUP) | Calories: 52 | Fat: 2 g | Protein: 1 g | Sodium: 10 mg | Fiber: <1 g | Carbohydrates: 6 g | Sugar: <1 g

Jumbo Pumpkin Chocolate Chip Muffins

Moist, dense, and pumpkin rich, these jumbo muffins are a meal in themselves.
Substitute chopped nuts or dried fruit for the chocolate chips if desired.

INGREDIENTS | YIELDS 6

1 cup pumpkin purée

⅔ cup light brown sugar

1 egg white

2 tablespoons canola oil

1 teaspoon pure vanilla extract

1 tablespoon sodium-free baking powder

½ teaspoon ground cinnamon

1 cup white whole-wheat flour

2 tablespoons low-fat milk

⅓ cup semisweet chocolate chips

1. Preheat oven to 400°F. Line a 6-cup jumbo muffin tin with paper liners and set aside.

2. Place the pumpkin, sugar, egg white, oil, and vanilla into a mixing bowl and stir well to combine. Add the remaining ingredients and mix until incorporated.

3. Spoon the batter into the tin, filling each cup about ⅔ full. Place pan on middle rack in oven and bake for 20–25 minutes.

4. Remove from oven and transfer muffins to a wire rack to cool.

PER SERVING (1 MUFFIN) | Calories: 287 | Fat: 8 g | Protein: 4 g | Sodium: 20 mg | Fiber: 3 g | Carbohydrates: 51 g | Sugar: 32 g

ABC Muffins

Apple, banana, and carrot give these muffins superb moistness and flavor. Packed with vitamins and nutrients, they make a great cholesterol-free breakfast or quick snack.

INGREDIENTS | YIELDS 1 DOZEN

2 medium apples, chopped

2 medium carrots, shredded

1 ripe medium banana, mashed

3 tablespoons canola oil

¼ cup nondairy milk

¼ cup brown sugar

1 tablespoon pure vanilla extract

1 cup unbleached all-purpose flour

¼ cup white whole-wheat flour

1½ teaspoons sodium-free baking powder

Sodium-Free Baking Powder

Standard baking powder, the kind typically sold in supermarkets, contains hundreds of mg of sodium per serving, and is not recommended on the DASH diet. Two brands of sodium-free baking powder are available and provide the same great rise in baked goods. Ener-G sodium-free baking powder can be purchased online. Featherweight sodium-free baking powder is sold online, at Whole Foods markets, and other select stores.

1. Preheat oven to 350°F. Spray a 12-muffin tin lightly with oil or line with paper liners. Set aside.

2. Place the apples, carrots, and banana into a bowl. Add the remaining ingredients and mix well.

3. Divide batter evenly among the muffin cups. Place tin on middle rack in oven and bake for 20–25 minutes.

4. Remove from oven and place tin on wire rack to cool. Cool fully before removing muffins from tin and eating.

PER SERVING (1 MUFFIN) | Calories: 128 | Fat: 4 g | Protein: 2 g | Sodium: 11 mg | Fiber: 2 g | Carbohydrates: 22 g | Sugar: 9 g

Whole-Wheat Strawberry Corn Muffins

Fabulous vegan muffins with the taste and texture of traditional. The combination of plump moist berries and subtle crunch of cornmeal is irresistible.

INGREDIENTS | YIELDS 1 DOZEN

1 cup white whole-wheat flour

½ cup cornmeal

½ cup sugar

1 tablespoon sodium-free baking powder

1 cup chopped fresh strawberries

1 cup nondairy milk

3 tablespoons canola oil

2 teaspoons pure vanilla extract

1. Preheat the oven to 375°F. Line a 12-cup muffin tin with paper liners and set aside.

2. Place the flour, cornmeal, sugar, and baking powder into a mixing bowl and whisk well to combine.

3. Add the strawberries, nondairy milk, oil, and vanilla and stir until incorporated.

4. Fill the muffin cups roughly ⅔ full. Place muffin tin on middle rack in oven and bake for 20 minutes.

5. Remove from oven and place on a wire rack to cool. Let muffins cool at least 10 minutes before serving to ensure paper wrappers come off with ease.

PER SERVING (1 MUFFIN) | Calories: 128 | Fat: 4 g | Protein: 2 g | Sodium: 10 mg | Fiber: 2 g | Carbohydrates: 21 g | Sugar: 9 g

Lemon Rhubarb Muffins

Sugar topped, moist, and yummy, these muffins are flecked with lemon zest and melt-in-your-mouth chunks of fruit.

INGREDIENTS | YIELDS 1 DOZEN

Egg replacement powder for 1 egg
1 cup diced fresh rhubarb
½ cup sugar
Juice and grated zest of 1 fresh lemon
¼ cup canola oil
1 tablespoon sodium-free baking powder
⅔ cup unbleached all-purpose flour
½ cup white whole-wheat flour
¼ cup nondairy milk
1 tablespoon demerara sugar

White Whole-Wheat Flour

Hard red wheat, the type of flour used in many whole-wheat breads, is high in nutrients, but its flavor can be overpowering. White whole-wheat flour has the same health benefits as red, but with a much lighter taste and texture. It can often be used interchangeably with all-purpose flour, and is a great way of boosting a recipe's fiber and nutrients without compromising taste. King Arthur Organic White Whole Wheat Flour is an excellent product, sold at many supermarkets and Whole Foods stores.

1. Preheat oven to 375°F. Line a 12-muffin tin with paper liners and set aside.

2. Prepare the egg replacement according to package directions.

3. Place the egg replacement, rhubarb, sugar, lemon juice, lemon zest, and oil into a mixing bowl and stir well to combine.

4. Add the baking powder and stir. Gradually add in the flours, then stir in the milk.

5. Divide the batter evenly between the muffin cups, filling about ⅔ full. Sprinkle ¼ teaspoon sugar on each muffin. Place pan on middle rack in oven and bake for 25 minutes.

6. Remove from oven and transfer to a wire rack to cool. Serve warm or cool.

PER SERVING (1 MUFFIN) | Calories: 132 | Fat: 5 g | Protein: 3 g | Sodium: 22 mg | Fiber: 1 g | Carbohydrates: 19 g | Sugar: 10 g

Crumb-Topped Mango Muffins

Let these warm tropical muffins remind you that paradise is just a state of mind. The soft vanilla-lemon crumb is dotted with juicy chunks of mango, and the tops explode out of the tin with the sweet crunch of macadamia nut crumbs.

INGREDIENTS | YIELDS 6

¼ cup brown sugar

¼ cup finely chopped unsalted macadamia nuts

1½ tablespoons unbleached all-purpose flour

½ teaspoon ground cinnamon

1 tablespoon unsalted butter

1½ cups unbleached all-purpose flour

½ cup white whole-wheat flour

1 tablespoon sodium-free baking powder

½ cup sugar

1 egg white

1 cup low-fat milk

3 tablespoons canola oil

1 teaspoon pure vanilla extract

Grated zest of 1 fresh lemon

1 fresh mango, peeled and finely diced

1. Preheat oven to 400°F. Spray a 6-cup jumbo muffin tin lightly with oil or line with disposable liners. Set aside.

2. First make the crumb topping. Combine the brown sugar, chopped nuts, flour, and cinnamon in a small mixing bowl. Cut the butter in with your fingertips, processing until it has the consistency of wet sand. Set aside.

3. To make the batter, measure the flours, baking powder, and sugar into a large mixing bowl and whisk well to combine.

4. Add the egg white, milk, oil, vanilla, and grated lemon zest and mix just until moist. Gently fold in the mango, stirring just until combined.

5. Fill the muffin cups about ¾ full, then top with the crumb mixture, dividing evenly between the cups (about 2 tablespoons each).

6. Place the pan on the middle rack in the oven and bake for 25–30 minutes. Remove from oven and gently move muffins to a wire rack to cool fully.

PER SERVING (1 MUFFIN) | Calories: 418 | Fat: 14 g | Protein: 7 g | Sodium: 32 mg | Fiber: 3 g | Carbohydrates: 67 g | Sugar: 33 g

Banana Nut Muffins

Sweet and moist with great banana flavor, the quintessential muffin gets a whole-grain makeover. Unbleached all-purpose flour may be used if you prefer.

INGREDIENTS | YIELDS 1 DOZEN

1 cup mashed banana

½ cup brown sugar

1 egg white

2 tablespoons canola oil

2 teaspoons pure vanilla extract

½ teaspoon ground cinnamon

2 teaspoons sodium-free baking powder

1½ cups white whole-wheat flour

1 tablespoon low-fat milk

¼ cup chopped walnuts

Baking with Bananas

Overripe, brown bananas may not be appealing to eat, but they lend fabulous flavor and enhanced sweetness to baked goods and smoothies, and may even eliminate the need for added sugar and oil. If you have overripe bananas on hand and don't have time to bake, seal them in a plastic bag or other container, and freeze for later use. Once frozen, the banana peels turn deep black, but the flesh inside remains perfectly fine and keeps for months.

1. Preheat oven to 375°F. Line a 12-muffin tin with paper liners and set aside.

2. In a mixing bowl, beat together the banana, brown sugar, egg white, oil, vanilla, and cinnamon.

3. Add the baking powder and stir well to combine. Gradually add in the flour, then the milk and walnuts. Stir until everything is incorporated.

4. Spoon batter into muffin cups, filling roughly ⅔ full. Place pan on middle rack in oven and bake for 18 minutes. Remove from oven and place on wire rack to cool.

PER SERVING (1 MUFFIN) | Calories: 143 | Fat: 4 g | Protein: 3 g | Sodium: 9 mg | Fiber: 2 g | Carbohydrates: 25 g | Sugar: 16 g

Jumbo Bakery-Style Muffins

Sure to become a favorite muffin. Subtly sweet, full of plump berries, with just a hint of lemon. Use whichever berries you like best, from fresh blueberries to raspberries, blackberries, strawberries, even pitted cherries.

INGREDIENTS | YIELDS 6

¼ cup brown sugar

1½ tablespoons unbleached all-purpose flour

½ teaspoon ground cinnamon

1 tablespoon unsalted butter

1½ cups unbleached all-purpose flour

½ cup white whole-wheat flour

1 tablespoon sodium-free baking powder

⅔ cup sugar

1 egg white

1 cup low-fat milk

¼ cup canola oil

1 teaspoon pure vanilla extract

1 teaspoon pure lemon extract

1¼ cups fresh berries

1. Preheat oven to 400°F. Grease a 6-cup jumbo muffin tin or line with disposable liners.

2. First make the crumb topping. Combine the brown sugar, flour, and cinnamon in a small mixing bowl. Cut the butter in with your (freshly washed) hands, processing until it has the consistency of wet sand. Set aside.

3. To make the batter, place the flours, baking powder, and sugar into a large mixing bowl and whisk well to combine.

4. Add the egg white, milk, oil, and extracts and mix just until moist. Gently fold in the berries, stirring just until combined.

5. Fill the muffin cups about ⅔ full, then top with the crumb mixture, dividing evenly between the cups.

6. Place the pan on the middle rack of the oven and bake for 20–25 minutes. Remove from oven and gently move muffins to a wire rack to cool fully.

PER SERVING (1 MUFFIN) | Calories: 414 | Fat: 12 g | Protein: 7 g | Sodium: 31 mg | Fiber: 3 g | Carbohydrates: 70 g | Sugar: 36 g

Maple, Oatmeal, Applesauce Muffins

Like a comforting bowl of oatmeal in a convenient package, these yummy muffins make any busy morning better. Bake a batch ahead of time, freeze, then pop one out the night before to thaw.

INGREDIENTS | YIELDS 1 DOZEN

1 cup low-fat milk
1 tablespoon distilled white vinegar
1 cup old-fashioned rolled oats
1 egg white
¼ cup canola oil
¼ cup unsweetened applesauce
⅓ cup brown sugar
¼ cup pure maple syrup
1 teaspoon ground cinnamon
2 teaspoons sodium-free baking powder
1 teaspoon sodium-free baking soda
1 cup unbleached all-purpose flour
¼ cup whole-wheat flour

Low-Sodium and Sodium-Free Products

The DASH diet requires you to purchase some specialty items, such as low-sodium baking powder and baking soda, that may not be available in local stores. Two online sources of these and many other low-sodium products are HealthyHeartMarket.com and HeartWiseFood.com.

1. Preheat oven to 425°F. Grease a 12-muffin tin or line with disposable liners. Set aside.

2. Pour the milk into a measuring glass and add the vinegar. Let sit 5 minutes.

3. Place the oats into a large mixing bowl; add the milk and let sit 10 minutes.

4. After the oats have softened, add the egg white, oil, and applesauce and stir well.

5. Add the brown sugar, maple syrup, and cinnamon and mix, then stir in the baking powder and baking soda.

6. Gradually add the flours, scraping the bowl well to combine.

7. Pour the batter into the muffin cups, dividing evenly. Place pan on the middle rack in the preheated oven and bake for 20–25 minutes. Muffins are done when tester inserted in center comes clean.

8. Remove pan from oven, then carefully remove muffins from cups and place on wire rack to cool.

PER SERVING (1 MUFFIN) | Calories: 164 | Fat: 5 g | Protein: 3 g | Sodium: 16 mg | Fiber: 1 g | Carbohydrates: 26 g | Sugar: 11 g

Zucchini Muffins

Here's a way to consume that bumper crop of zucchini. These moist muffins are absolutely delicious and freeze beautifully, so you can bake several batches to enjoy in colder weather.

INGREDIENTS | YIELDS 1 DOZEN

1¼ cups shredded zucchini

2 egg whites

⅔ cup sugar

⅓ cup canola oil

2 teaspoons pure vanilla extract

1 teaspoon ground cinnamon

¼ teaspoon ground nutmeg

2 teaspoons sodium-free baking powder

1 cup unbleached all-purpose flour

½ cup white whole-wheat flour

¼ cup chopped walnuts

¼ cup seedless raisins

1. Preheat oven to 350°F. Spray a 12-muffin tin lightly with oil or line with paper liners. Set aside.

2. Place zucchini into a mixing bowl and add the egg whites, sugar, oil, vanilla, cinnamon, and nutmeg. Stir well.

3. Add the baking powder and stir. Add in the flours, then the walnuts and raisins, and stir just until combined.

4. Divide batter evenly between the muffin cups. Place pan on middle rack in oven and bake for 20–30 minutes. Muffins are done when tester inserted in center comes clean.

5. Remove pan from oven and place on wire rack to cool.

PER SERVING (1 MUFFIN) | Calories: 183 | Fat: 7 g | Protein: 3 g | Sodium: 11 mg | Fiber: 1 g | Carbohydrates: 26 g | Sugar: 13 g

Chocolate-Chocolate Chip Banana Muffins

*Moist and dense, these double-chocolate muffins are full of hearty
whole-grain goodness and subtle banana flavor.*

INGREDIENTS | YIELDS 1 DOZEN

3 medium bananas, mashed

3 tablespoons canola oil

⅓ cup unsweetened cocoa powder

⅓ cup brown sugar

1 tablespoon sodium-free baking powder

1 cup white whole-wheat flour

1 egg white

½ cup low-fat milk

¼ cup semisweet chocolate chips

Regular Flour Versus Pastry Flour

What's the difference between pastry flour and regular flour? Simply the fineness of the grain. Substitute whole-wheat pastry flour (sometimes called graham flour) for standard whole wheat to achieve a much finer, lighter crumb in your cookies, muffins, and cakes. Pastry flour is not recommended for use in traditional bread recipes.

1. Preheat oven to 350°F. Line a standard 12-cup muffin tin with paper liners or spray lightly with oil and flour. Set aside.

2. Place all of the ingredients into a mixing bowl and stir well to combine.

3. Pour batter into the prepared muffin tin, filling cups about ⅔ full. Place pan on middle rack in oven and bake for 20 minutes.

4. Remove from oven and transfer to a wire rack to cool. Cool at least 10 minutes before serving to ensure paper liners release easily from muffins.

PER SERVING (1 MUFFIN) | Calories: 156 | Fat: 5 g | Protein: 4 g | Sodium: 50 mg | Fiber: 2 g | Carbohydrates: 25 g | Sugar: 12 g

Pumpkin Cranberry Scones

*Beautifully delicious and easy to make,
these tasty scones are perfect for fall mornings.*

INGREDIENTS | YIELDS 8

2⅓ cups white whole-wheat flour

½ cup light brown sugar

4 teaspoons sodium-free baking powder

6 tablespoons unsalted butter

½ cup low-fat milk

1 cup pumpkin purée

¼ cup dried cranberries

1 teaspoon demerara sugar

Pumpkin Facts

Pumpkins are a type of winter squash with a hard outer shell and firm inner flesh. Like all winter squash, pumpkins must be cooked before eating. To prepare a pie pumpkin, simply cut in half, remove the seeds, and place halves in a microwave-safe bowl. Add an inch or two of water and microwave on high roughly 20 minutes. Scoop out cooked purée and use as desired, or freeze for later use. Pumpkin is an excellent source of vitamins A and C and fiber.

1. Preheat oven to 425°F. Line a baking sheet with parchment and set aside.

2. Place the flour, brown sugar, and baking powder into a mixing bowl and whisk well to combine.

3. Cut the butter into small pieces and work into the mixture using your (freshly washed) hands. Once the mixture resembles coarse crumbs, stir in the milk, pumpkin, and cranberries.

4. Turn the dough out onto a lightly floured surface and pat into a large round, roughly 9 inches in diameter. Using a long, sharp knife, cut the dough across into 8 equal wedges. Transfer wedges to the baking sheet. Sprinkle the tops of the scones with the demerara sugar.

5. Place pan on middle rack in oven and bake for 15 minutes. Remove from oven and transfer scones to a wire rack to cool.

PER SERVING | Calories: 274 | Fat: 9 g | Protein: 5 g | Sodium: 15 mg | Fiber: 5 g | Carbohydrates: 45 g | Sugar: 18 g

Lemon Coconut Scones

Light and sweet, these lovely lemon-scented scones are made for a special occasion. Like today!

INGREDIENTS | YIELDS 8

2 cups unbleached all-purpose flour

⅔ cup sugar

1 tablespoon sodium-free baking powder

5 tablespoons unsalted butter

5 ounces light coconut milk

Juice and grated zest of 1 fresh lemon

1. Preheat oven to 425°F. Line a baking sheet with parchment and set aside.

2. Measure the flour, sugar, and baking powder into a mixing bowl and whisk well to combine.

3. Cut the butter into small pieces and work into the mixture using your (freshly washed) hands. Once the mixture resembles coarse crumbs, stir in the coconut milk, lemon juice, and grated zest.

4. Turn the dough out onto a lightly floured surface and pat into a large round, roughly 9 inches in diameter. Using a long, sharp knife, cut the dough across into 8 equal wedges. Transfer wedges to the baking sheet.

5. Place pan on middle rack in oven and bake for 12 minutes. Remove from oven and transfer scones to a wire rack to cool.

PER SERVING | Calories: 255 | Fat: 8 g | Protein: 3 g | Sodium: 5 mg | Fiber: 1 g | Carbohydrates: 40 g | Sugar: 17 g

CHAPTER 4

Breakfasts

Swiss Cheese and Chive Mini Quiches

These tasty treats look impressive, but require very little preparation and equipment—all you need is a rolling pin and muffin tin. Feel free to vary the ingredients according to mood and season.

INGREDIENTS | YIELDS 1 DOZEN

¾ cup unbleached all-purpose flour

½ teaspoon salt-free all-purpose seasoning

¼ teaspoon dried dill

2 tablespoons unsalted butter

Water, as needed

2 eggs

⅔ cup low-fat milk

⅓ cup nonfat or low-fat sour cream

2 tablespoons all-purpose flour

6 tablespoons shredded Swiss cheese

¼ cup chopped fresh chives

Freshly ground black pepper, to taste

1. Preheat oven to 350°F. Take out a 12-cup muffin tin and set aside.

2. To make the crust, measure ¾ cup flour, seasoning, and dill into a mixing bowl and whisk to combine. Cut the butter into the mixture using your hands, processing until a fine crumb has been achieved.

3. Add cold water, ½ tablespoon at a time, until the dough just comes together. Roll the dough out thinly and cut into 12 (roughly) 2-inch circles using a biscuit cutter or drinking glass. Lightly spray the muffin tin with oil and line each cup with a round of dough.

4. To prepare the filling, beat the eggs, milk, sour cream, and 2 tablespoons flour in a mixing bowl until well combined.

5. Divide mixture evenly between the muffin tins. Top each with ½ tablespoon shredded Swiss cheese and 1 teaspoon of fresh chives. Sprinkle with freshly ground black pepper to taste.

6. Place pan on middle rack in oven and bake for 25 minutes. Remove from oven and let rest for a few minutes. Remove mini quiches by sliding a knife around edges and gently lifting up. Serve warm or at room temperature.

PER SERVING (2 MINI QUICHES) | Calories: 170 | Fat: 7 g | Protein: 7 g | Sodium: 93 mg | Fiber: 1 g | Carbohydrates: 18 g | Sugar: 2 g

Homemade Sausage Patties

This delicious homemade sausage is scented with sage and has a nice red pepper kick. Welcome back to breakfast, low-sodium dieters!

INGREDIENTS | SERVES 8

2 pounds lean ground pork
1 egg white
2 teaspoons brown sugar
2½ teaspoons ground sage
1 teaspoon dried marjoram
¾ teaspoon dried red pepper flakes
½ teaspoon freshly ground black pepper
¼ teaspoon ground rosemary

1. Combine ingredients in a large bowl and mix well using a fork or your hands. Form mixture into 16 (roughly) 2-inch patties.

2. Heat griddle or skillet over medium and brown patties on both sides, about 5 minutes per side. Lower heat to medium-low or low if they seem to be burning. Drain on paper towels before serving.

PER SERVING | Calories: 186 | Fat: 9 g | Protein: 22 g | Sodium: 67 mg | Fiber: 0 g | Carbohydrates: 1 g | Sugar: 1 g

Get Creative!

Homemade sausage isn't simply for breakfast. Sausage makes a terrific topping for pizza, adds spice and interest to plain pasta and sauce, and elevates boring meatloaf to something special. Double the batch whenever you make sausage, and freeze leftover patties for use in future recipes.

Maple Turkey Sausage

Perfect for those avoiding pork or simply looking for another lean breakfast meat. These homemade patties are subtly sweet and absolutely delicious.

INGREDIENTS | SERVES 8

2 pounds lean ground turkey
1 egg white
1 tablespoon pure maple syrup
1 tablespoon ground sage
½ teaspoon dried red pepper flakes
½ teaspoon fennel seed
½ teaspoon freshly ground black pepper
½ teaspoon ground rosemary
¼ teaspoon garlic powder

1. Combine ingredients in a large bowl and mix well using a fork or your hands. The mixture will be sticky. Form into 16 (roughly) 2-inch patties.

2. Heat griddle or skillet over medium and brown patties on both sides, about 4 minutes per side. Lower heat to medium-low or low if they seem to be burning. Drain on paper towels before serving.

PER SERVING | Calories: 161 | Fat: 7 g | Protein: 22 g | Sodium: 87 mg | Fiber: 0 g | Carbohydrates: 1 g | Sugar: 1 g

Scrambled Tofu with Mushrooms, Peppers, and Tomatoes

This is a great salt-free dish, especially good for vegans or those watching their cholesterol, and the taste is surprisingly authentic. Adapted from a recipe by Christina Pirello. Many thanks to Christa for passing it along!

INGREDIENTS | SERVES 4

1 small onion, diced

1 clove garlic, minced

1 cup sliced mushrooms

1 small tomato, diced

1 small bell pepper, diced

1 pound firm or extra-firm tofu, drained

½ teaspoon all-purpose salt-free seasoning

½ teaspoon freshly ground black pepper, or to taste

½ teaspoon ground turmeric

1. Place a nonstick skillet over medium heat. Add the onion, garlic, mushrooms, tomato, and bell pepper and cook, stirring, for 5 minutes.

2. Crumble the tofu over top, keeping it in rather large chunks. Add the salt-free seasoning, black pepper, and turmeric, and stir gently to combine. Cook another 5 minutes, stirring gently.

3. Remove from heat and serve immediately.

PER SERVING | Calories: 124 | Fat: 6 g | Protein: 12 g | Sodium: 7 mg | Fiber: 2 g | Carbohydrates: 6 g | Sugar: 1 g

What Is Turmeric?

Turmeric is a spice made from the ground root of the turmeric plant. Its bright yellow color and distinct flavor are used in many types of food, from Indian cuisine to prepared mustard. Turmeric has a slightly bitter taste that works well in combination with other seasonings. It's high in manganese and iron, and may help reduce the risk of some cancers.

Scrambled Eggs with Apples, Sage, and Swiss

This combination of tastes and textures seems tailor made for fall. The warmth and softness of the eggs, the tang of the Swiss, the play of apple against shallot, and the sage—don't forget the sage! That woodsy scent draws everything together.

INGREDIENTS | SERVES 2

2 eggs

1 medium apple, cored and chopped

1 shallot, chopped

¼ cup shredded Swiss cheese

1 teaspoon chopped fresh sage (or ½ teaspoon dried sage)

Freshly ground black pepper, to taste

1. Break eggs into a small bowl and beat well; set aside.

2. Place a nonstick skillet over medium-low heat. Add the chopped apple and shallot and cook, stirring, until soft but not brown, roughly 3–5 minutes.

3. Add the beaten egg. Let set roughly 30 seconds, then cook, stirring, 30 seconds to 1 minute more, until egg is almost cooked. Add Swiss cheese and stir.

4. Remove from heat and serve immediately, sprinkled with sage and freshly ground black pepper to taste.

PER SERVING | Calories: 165 | Fat: 8 g | Protein: 10 g | Sodium: 97 mg | Fiber: 2 g | Carbohydrates: 12 g | Sugar: 8 g

Diner-Style Home Fries

Tender, seasoned potatoes sautéed with onion and bell pepper.
This makes the most delicious side dish at breakfast. Enjoy leftovers later in the day!

INGREDIENTS | SERVES 6

4 medium potatoes, cut into ½-inch cubes
1 teaspoon olive oil
1 medium onion, diced
1 medium sweet bell pepper, diced
1 tablespoon salt-free tomato paste
2 teaspoons ground sweet paprika
½ teaspoon dried thyme
½ teaspoon garlic powder
½ teaspoon ground rosemary
¼ teaspoon freshly ground black pepper

1. Place diced potato into a microwave-safe bowl and cover with plastic wrap. Microwave for 7 minutes.

2. While potato is cooking, heat oil in a nonstick skillet over medium. Add onion and bell pepper and cook, stirring, for 7 minutes.

3. Add cooked potatoes to skillet, along with tomato paste and seasonings. Stir to combine, then cook, stirring, another 2–3 minutes. Remove from heat and serve.

PER SERVING | Calories: 101 | Fat: 1 g | Protein: 2 g | Sodium: 10 mg | Fiber: 2 g | Carbohydrates: 21 g | Sugar: 2 g

Variations on a Theme

Home fries and hashes make an easy and inexpensive breakfast and can be crafted using almost anything. Instead of standard potatoes, try making home fries with sweet potatoes, crumbled low-sodium bacon, and leeks. Dice leftover meat, hard-boiled eggs, and/or low-sodium cheese and add to the mix. Or shred a big variety of vegetables and make yourself a super vegan hash.

30-Minute Breakfast Pizza

Adapted from an old Pillsbury recipe for a modern, low-sodium audience. This fabulous pizza makes any breakfast into a party! Top with sliced tomatoes and fresh herbs if desired. Unbleached all-purpose or gluten-free flour may be used instead.

INGREDIENTS | SERVES 8

1 cup white whole-wheat flour

1 teaspoon all-purpose salt-free seasoning

1 teaspoon dried Italian seasoning

½ teaspoon garlic powder

Freshly ground black pepper, to taste

2 egg whites

⅔ cup low-fat milk

½ pound lean ground pork or turkey

1 teaspoon light brown sugar

½ teaspoon dried marjoram

¼ teaspoon dried red pepper flakes

¼ teaspoon freshly ground black pepper

¼ teaspoon ground sage

⅛ teaspoon ground rosemary

1 small onion, diced

2 eggs, beaten

½ cup shredded Swiss cheese

Learning to Live Low Sodium

It's hard to change the way you eat overnight; doubly challenging if you're preparing meals for a family. During difficult transitions, remind yourself and others of the reasons for change. Food is nourishment, but it can also be regarded as medicine. You are what you eat. The DASH diet offers a lifeline of health to you and your family; one of the greatest gifts you can give.

1. Preheat oven to 425°F. Grease and flour a 12-inch pizza pan and set aside.

2. Measure the flour into a mixing bowl. Add the salt-free seasoning, Italian seasoning, garlic powder, and freshly ground black pepper to taste and whisk well to combine.

3. Add the egg whites and milk and mix well. Pour batter onto the prepared pizza pan and spread to even.

4. In a large bowl, mix the ground meat with the brown sugar, marjoram, red pepper flakes, black pepper, sage, and rosemary.

5. Heat a skillet over medium, add seasoned meat and onion, and cook until browned, about 5 minutes. Drain any excess fat.

6. Sprinkle the meat and onion mixture evenly over the batter. Place pan on middle rack in oven and bake for 20 minutes.

7. While crust is baking, heat a nonstick skillet over medium-low. Add beaten eggs and let sit for roughly 30 seconds to set, then using a heatproof spatula or wooden spoon, gently stir the eggs until fully cooked, roughly 2 minutes. Remove from heat.

8. Remove pan from oven. Top baked pizza with scrambled egg and cheese. Return pan to oven for 3 minutes. Remove pizza and cut into slices. Serve immediately.

PER SERVING | Calories: 145 | Fat: 5 g | Protein: 12 g | Sodium: 72 mg | Fiber: 2 g | Carbohydrates: 13 g | Sugar: 2 g

Homemade Granola

Subtly sweet and super crunchy, this cereal keeps well for weeks when stored in an airtight container. The dried fruit is stirred in after the cereal has fully cooled, so it stays soft. Unsweetened shredded coconut lends a lot of flavor without much sodium; eliminate if you're watching your fat.

INGREDIENTS | YIELDS 10 CUPS

6 cups quick or old-fashioned oats

1¼ cups unsalted chopped nuts (your choice)

½ cup dried unsweetened coconut

1 teaspoon ground cinnamon

½ teaspoon ground ginger

¼ teaspoon ground cloves

¼ teaspoon ground nutmeg

1 cup pure maple syrup

1½ tablespoons pure vanilla extract

2 cups chopped dried fruit (your choice)

1. Preheat oven to 350°F. Take out 2 sided baking sheets, spray lightly with oil, and set aside.

2. In a large mixing bowl, combine the oats, chopped nuts, shredded coconut, cinnamon, ginger, cloves, and nutmeg.

3. Add the maple syrup and vanilla and stir until everything is thoroughly coated.

4. Divide the mixture between the 2 baking sheets. Place sheets on middle rack in oven and bake until golden brown, roughly 25–30 minutes. Two or three times during baking, remove pans from oven and carefully stir contents before returning to oven. This will ensure even baking so granola does not burn.

5. Once golden, remove pans from oven and set aside to cool fully. Once fully cooled, stir the dried fruit into the mixture. Store in an airtight container.

PER SERVING | Calories: 266 | Fat: 10 g | Protein: 5 g | Sodium: 7 mg | Fiber: 4 g | Carbohydrates: 42 g | Sugar: 19 g

5-Spice Quinoa with Apples and Raisins

A simple, hot, and filling breakfast especially great in fall and winter. Keep the peel on the apple for added nutrients and fiber. If you prefer softer fruit, add during cooking time rather than after.

INGREDIENTS | SERVES 4

1 cup uncooked quinoa
1 cup water
1 cup unsweetened apple juice
½ teaspoon ground 5-spice powder
1 medium apple, chopped
¼ cup seedless raisins

1. Measure quinoa, water, apple juice, and 5-spice powder into a saucepan. Bring to a boil over high heat.

2. Once boiling, reduce heat to medium-low, cover pot, and simmer for 15 minutes.

3. Remove from heat, stir in apple and raisins, and serve immediately.

PER SERVING | Calories: 207 | Fat: 2 g | Protein: 5 g | Sodium: 11 mg | Fiber: 4 g | Carbohydrates: 43 g | Sugar: 16 g

Saturday Morning Pancakes

Weekends were made for hot, fluffy pancakes. This tried-and-true recipe is great with any type of flour, and can be adapted for vegans by using nondairy milk and egg replacement powder.

INGREDIENTS | SERVES 4

1⅓ cups white whole-wheat flour
¼ cup sugar
1 tablespoon sodium-free baking powder
1½ cups low-fat milk
1 egg white
1 tablespoon canola oil
1 tablespoon pure vanilla extract

1. Measure the flour, sugar, and baking powder into a mixing bowl and whisk well to combine.

2. Add the milk, egg, oil, and vanilla. Mix well and let sit for 1–2 minutes to thicken.

3. Place nonstick griddle or skillet on stove and turn heat to medium. Pour batter onto heated griddle. When pancake has bubbled on top and is nicely browned on bottom (approximately 2–4 minutes), flip over. Brown on second side another 2–3 minutes. If pancakes are browning too quickly, lower heat.

4. Repeat process with remaining batter. Serve pancakes warm.

PER SERVING | Calories: 266 | Fat: 5 g | Protein: 9 g | Sodium: 56 mg | Fiber: 4 g | Carbohydrates: 46 g | Sugar: 17 g

Breakfast on the Go!

Life on a low-sodium diet can be inconvenient. Save yourself hunger and hassle by doubling pancake or waffle recipes on the weekends. Place leftovers between small sheets of waxed paper, store in plastic bags, and freeze. A frozen pancake or waffle will defrost in minutes.

Yogurt Parfaits

Healthy, filling, and well-balanced, this breakfast is more of a suggestion than a recipe per se.
Feel free to embellish according to season and personal preference.

INGREDIENTS | SERVES 2

1 cup low-fat yogurt
1 ripe banana, peeled and sliced
½ cup fresh blueberries
¼ cup low-fat, low-sodium granola

1. Spoon yogurt evenly into 2 small bowls or glasses, top with fruit and cereal.

2. Serve immediately.

PER SERVING | Calories: 208 | Fat: 3 g | Protein: 8 g | Sodium: 58 mg | Fiber: 2 g | Carbohydrates: 38 g | Sugar: 20 g

Breakfast Cereal Alert

Breakfast cereals are highly processed foods and often contain large quantities of sodium. Before selecting a cereal, it's important to check the nutrition facts carefully. Just because a cereal contains whole grains does not necessarily make it good for you. Many supposedly healthy cereals contain more than 140 mg of sodium per serving. Read nutrition labels; don't believe the hype.

Brown Sugar Cinnamon Oatmeal

A sweet and creamy oatmeal as delicious as those instant packets, but without the high sodium and artificial additives. And only 5 minutes from start to finish; it's a win-win you're sure to love.

INGREDIENTS | SERVES 4

2 cups low-fat milk
1½ teaspoons pure vanilla extract
1⅓ cups quick oats
¼ cup light brown sugar
½ teaspoon ground cinnamon

1. Measure the milk and vanilla into a medium saucepan and bring to a boil over medium-high heat.

2. Once boiling, reduce heat to medium, stir in oats, brown sugar, and cinnamon, and cook, stirring, 2–3 minutes.

3. Serve immediately, sprinkled with additional cinnamon if desired.

PER SERVING | Calories: 208 | Fat: 3 g | Protein: 8 g | Sodium: 58 mg | Fiber: 2 g | Carbohydrates: 38 g | Sugar: 20 g

Coconut Rice with Dried Apricots and Mint

This sweet rice makes a scrumptious hot alternative to oatmeal. Omit the agave nectar if you prefer it less sweet. Try adding chopped nuts and serving as a side dish with a later meal.

INGREDIENTS | SERVES 4

¾ cup light coconut milk

¼ cup water

½ cup basmati rice, rinsed well

1 tablespoon agave nectar (optional)

⅓ cup dried apricots, diced

⅛ teaspoon ground cardamom

1 tablespoon chopped fresh mint

1. Combine the coconut milk and water in a 3-quart saucepan. Bring to a boil over high heat.

2. Once boiling, add the rice, reduce heat to low, cover, and simmer for 15 minutes.

3. Remove pot from heat. Stir in the agave nectar, dried apricots, cardamom, and mint. Serve immediately.

PER SERVING | Calories: 118 | Fat: 3 g | Protein: 1 g | Sodium: 10 mg | Fiber: 1 g | Carbohydrates: 20 g | Sugar: 8 g

What Is Agave Nectar?

Agave nectar is a liquid sweetener derived from the agave cactus. It's a clear, light brown liquid, similar in look to maple syrup, though slightly thicker. It has a subtle pleasant flavor, and is very sweet, about twice as sweet as cane sugar. Because of its liquid form, it dissolves instantly, making it a great choice for sweetening beverages and dressings. Unlike honey, agave nectar is a strictly vegan food.

Hot Honey Porridge

Warm and filling, this healthy multigrain cereal has a soft honey taste and a creamy, slightly chewy texture. Add dried fruit or chopped nuts if desired.

INGREDIENTS | SERVES 4

¾ cup bulgur wheat

½ cup rolled oats

3 cups boiling water

¼ cup honey

1. Place the bulgur and oats into a saucepan. Add the boiling water and stir to combine.

2. Place pan over high heat and bring to a boil. Once boiling, reduce heat to low, cover, and simmer for 10 minutes, stirring occasionally.

3. Remove from heat, stir in honey, and serve immediately.

PER SERVING | Calories: 172 | Fat: 1 g | Protein: 4 g | Sodium: 5 mg | Fiber: 5 g | Carbohydrates: 40 g | Sugar: 17 g

Whole-Wheat Cinnamon Pancakes with Banana

These scrumptious pancakes, flavored with ripe banana, cinnamon, and vanilla, make a fabulous low-fat breakfast.

INGREDIENTS | SERVES 4

1⅓ cups white whole-wheat flour

¼ cup sugar

1 tablespoon sodium-free baking powder

1⅓ cups low-fat milk

1 egg white

1 teaspoon ground cinnamon

1 tablespoon pure vanilla extract

1 ripe banana, sliced

1. Measure the flour, sugar, and baking powder into a mixing bowl and whisk well to combine.

2. Add the milk, egg white, cinnamon, and vanilla. Mix well and let sit for 1–2 minutes to thicken.

3. Place nonstick griddle or skillet on stove and turn heat to medium. Pour batter onto heated griddle. Arrange ¼ of the banana slices over top. When pancake has bubbled on top and is nicely browned on bottom (approximately 2–4 minutes), flip over. Brown on second side another 2–3 minutes. If pancakes are browning too quickly, lower heat.

4. Repeat process with remaining batter. Serve pancakes warm.

PER SERVING | Calories: 274 | Fat: 1 g | Protein: 9 g | Sodium: 53 mg | Fiber: 6 g | Carbohydrates: 54 g | Sugar: 21 g

Chocolate Pancakes

Make any morning feel like a special occasion. Add white chocolate chips, dried cranberries, or chopped nuts to the batter for an extra-special treat.

INGREDIENTS | SERVES 4

1 cup white whole-wheat flour

¼ cup unsweetened cocoa powder

¼ cup sugar

1 tablespoon sodium-free baking powder

1½ cups low-fat milk

1 egg

2 tablespoons canola oil

½ teaspoon pure vanilla extract

1. Measure the flour, cocoa powder, sugar, and baking powder into a mixing bowl and whisk well to combine.

2. Add the milk, egg, oil, and vanilla. Mix well.

3. Place nonstick griddle or skillet on stove and turn heat to medium. Pour batter onto heated griddle. When pancake has bubbled on top and is nicely browned on bottom (approximately 2–4 minutes), flip over. Brown on second side another 2–3 minutes. If pancakes are browning too quickly, lower heat.

4. Repeat process with remaining batter. Serve pancakes warm, with whipped cream and real maple syrup if desired.

PER SERVING | Calories: 251 | Fat: 7 g | Protein: 9 g | Sodium: 60 mg | Fiber: 5 g | Carbohydrates: 42 g | Sugar: 17 g

From Soup to . . . Pancakes?

Soup ladles aren't just for soup. They work wonderfully for measuring and pouring pancake batter onto any hot cooking surface. The resulting pancakes will be perfectly shaped and sized, and you'll never worry about messy cleanup! Ladles work wonderfully when measuring waffle batter, too.

Oven-Baked Apple Pancake

A light and fluffy pancake made without milk and eggs? It's true! Moist, airy, and delicious, this cholesterol-free pancake will impress with its taste and simplicity. Just whisk together the ingredients, pour, and bake. The oven does all of the work.

INGREDIENTS | SERVES 8

2 cups diced apple

1 tablespoon pure vanilla extract

1 tablespoon sodium-free baking powder

1 cup unbleached all-purpose flour

⅓ cup unsweetened applesauce

⅓ cup real maple syrup

¾ cup nondairy milk

1 tablespoon sugar

½ teaspoon ground cinnamon

Choices, Choices

There's a nondairy milk for every taste. From soy and rice milks to almond, coconut, hemp, oat, and more. Plain, sweetened, even flavored varieties exist. Don't know which to try? Sample different brands, varieties, and flavors until you find one or more you enjoy. You can even make your own nondairy milk at home. It's not hard, but is best made using a super-strong blender, such as Vitamix.

1. Preheat oven to 400°F. Lightly spray an ovenproof skillet with oil.

2. Place the apple, vanilla, baking powder, flour, applesauce, maple syrup, and nondairy milk into a large mixing bowl and stir well to combine. Pour batter into the prepared skillet and smooth top to even.

3. Combine the sugar and cinnamon in a small bowl and sprinkle evenly over the batter.

4. Place pan on middle rack in oven and bake for 25 minutes. Remove from oven. Carefully loosen pancake from pan using a spatula. Slice into sections and serve immediately.

PER SERVING | Calories: 126 | Fat: 1 g | Protein: 2 g | Sodium: 10 mg | Fiber: 1 g | Carbohydrates: 27 g | Sugar: 13 g

Orange Cornmeal Pancakes

Wake up with bright citrus and a moist corn crunch.
These light, fluffy pancakes are so good, you may even pass on the syrup.

INGREDIENTS | SERVES 4

⅔ cup white whole-wheat flour

⅔ cup cornmeal

1 tablespoon sodium-free baking powder

¼ cup sugar

3 tablespoons freshly squeezed orange juice

1½ teaspoons minced orange zest

1 cup low-fat milk

1 egg white

1. Measure all the ingredients into a mixing bowl and stir well to combine.

2. Place nonstick griddle or skillet on stove and turn heat to medium-low. Pour batter onto heated griddle. When pancake has bubbled on top and is nicely browned on bottom, roughly 2 minutes, flip over. Brown on second side, roughly 2 minutes more. If pancakes are browning too quickly, lower heat.

3. Repeat process with remaining batter. Serve immediately.

PER SERVING | Calories: 223 | Fat: 2 g | Protein: 7 g | Sodium: 48 mg | Fiber: 4 g | Carbohydrates: 46 g | Sugar: 16 g

Sweet Potato Breakfast Pie

A cross between hash browns and a pancake, this super-healthy oven-baked breakfast
will garner rave reviews. Serve plain or drizzled lightly with maple syrup.

INGREDIENTS | SERVES 8

2 cups shredded sweet potato

1 cup shredded carrot

¼ cup white whole-wheat flour

2 egg whites

1 tablespoon pure maple syrup

1 tablespoon freshly squeezed orange juice

½ teaspoon minced orange zest

¼ teaspoon ground cinnamon

1. Preheat oven to 425°F. Spray a pie pan lightly with oil and set aside.

2. Place all the ingredients into a mixing bowl and stir well to combine. Spread mixture in the prepared pan and smooth top to even.

3. Place pan on middle rack in oven and bake for 20 minutes. Remove from oven and cut into wedges. Serve warm.

PER SERVING | Calories: 75 | Fat: 4 g | Protein: 2 g | Sodium: 41 mg | Fiber: 2 g | Carbohydrates: 16 g | Sugar: 5 g

Sunday Morning Waffles

Homemade waffles are such a simple, yet impressive breakfast. As a bonus, they freeze beautifully, so you can make them in bulk, store them in the freezer, then toast for quick weekday breakfasts.

INGREDIENTS | SERVES 6

1⅔ cups unbleached all-purpose flour
¼ cup sugar
1 tablespoon sodium-free baking powder
2 egg whites
1½ cups low-fat milk
2 teaspoons pure vanilla extract
2 tablespoons canola oil

Waffle Tip

After removing waffles from the waffle iron, place directly on the middle rack of a preheated 200°F oven, bake 5 minutes, remove, and serve. When serving, do not stack the waffles. The moisture from the waffles will condense and cause waffles to become limp. Always serve waffles in a single layer to keep them fresh and crisp.

1. Place flour, sugar, and baking powder into a mixing bowl and whisk well to combine.

2. Place egg whites into another mixing bowl and beat until they form stiff peaks.

3. Add milk, vanilla, and canola oil to the dry ingredients and mix well. Let rest for 1–2 minutes to thicken, then gently fold whites into the batter.

4. Heat waffle iron. Spray lightly with oil, then ladle batter onto the hot surface, being careful to avoid the edges (batter will spread once appliance is closed). Close waffle iron and bake until golden brown, roughly 4–5 minutes.

5. Remove baked waffles from iron and repeat process with remaining batter. Serve immediately.

PER SERVING | Calories: 220 | Fat: 6 g | Protein: 7 g | Sodium: 46 mg | Fiber: 4 g | Carbohydrates: 35 g | Sugar: 11 g

Whole-Grain Spiced Pear Waffles

*Crisp and hearty, these healthy waffles
are also great with chopped apple and walnuts.*

INGREDIENTS | SERVES 8

1 medium pear

1⅔ cups white whole-wheat flour

⅓ cup sugar

1½ tablespoons sodium-free baking powder

2 cups low-fat milk

1 egg white

2 tablespoons canola oil

2 teaspoons pure vanilla extract

1 teaspoon ground cinnamon

½ teaspoon ground ginger

¼ teaspoon ground nutmeg

1. Peel, core, and finely chop the pear. Place into a mixing bowl, add remaining ingredients, and beat until smooth.

2. Heat waffle iron. Spray lightly with oil, then ladle batter onto the hot surface, being careful to avoid the edges (batter will spread once appliance is closed). Close waffle iron and bake until golden brown, roughly 4–5 minutes.

3. Remove baked waffles from iron and repeat process with remaining batter. Serve immediately.

PER SERVING | Calories: 192 | Fat: 4 g | Protein: 6 g | Sodium: 35 mg | Fiber: 4 g | Carbohydrates: 33 g | Sugar: 14 g

Pumpkin Waffles

Everything's better with pumpkin! This super breakfast is packed with healthy whole grain and vitamin A.

INGREDIENTS | SERVES 6

1 cup pumpkin purée

1 cup white whole-wheat flour

½ cup unbleached all-purpose flour

⅓ cup brown sugar

1½ cups low-fat milk

1 egg white

1 tablespoon canola oil

1 tablespoon sodium-free baking powder

1 tablespoon pure vanilla extract

2 teaspoons ground cinnamon

¼ teaspoon ground allspice

¼ teaspoon ground ginger

1. Measure ingredients into a large mixing bowl and beat until smooth.

2. Heat waffle iron. Spray lightly with oil, then ladle batter onto the hot surface, being careful to avoid the edges (batter will spread once appliance is closed). Close waffle iron and bake until golden brown, roughly 4–5 minutes.

3. Remove baked waffles from iron and repeat process with remaining batter. Serve immediately.

PER SERVING | Calories: 219 | Fat: 3 g | Protein: 7 g | Sodium: 43 mg | Fiber: 4 g | Carbohydrates: 41 g | Sugar: 16 g

Baked Doughnuts

The recipe below yields a dozen delicious cinnamon-sugar doughnuts. Skip the last step in the recipe to serve them plain. Doughnuts are also great glazed, frosted, or dusted with powdered sugar.

INGREDIENTS | YIELDS 1 DOZEN

2 cups white whole-wheat flour

⅔ cup sugar

1 tablespoon sodium-free baking powder

1 teaspoon ground cinnamon

1 cup low-fat milk

1 teaspoon pure vanilla extract

2 egg whites

2 tablespoons sugar

¾ teaspoon ground cinnamon

2 tablespoons unsalted butter, melted

Doughnut Pans

Doughnuts pans, like muffins tins, are metal trays with special circular cutouts for batter. In the case of a doughnut pan, however, the rounds are wide and shallow, with a small tubular protrusion in the center for the doughnut hole. Doughnut pans are inexpensive and will last for years if gently hand washed. Select a pan with a nonstick coating to minimize the need for added oil. Doughnut pans are sold at kitchen stores, big box retailers, and other locations.

1. Preheat oven to 425°F. Lightly spray a doughnut pan with oil and set aside.

2. Measure the flour, sugar, baking powder, and cinnamon into a mixing bowl and whisk to combine.

3. Add the milk, vanilla, and egg whites and beat well.

4. Spoon batter into doughnut pan, filling about ⅔ full.

5. Place pan on middle rack in oven and bake for 10 minutes. Remove pan from oven and let rest a few minutes before gently removing doughnuts from pan.

6. Measure the sugar and cinnamon into a small bowl and mix to combine. Dip doughnuts quickly in melted butter and sprinkle with cinnamon-sugar mixture.

7. Serve immediately or place on wire rack to cool.

PER SERVING (1 DOUGHNUT) | Calories: 147 | Fat: 2 g | Protein: 4 g | Sodium: 19 mg | Fiber: 2 g | Carbohydrates: 28 g | Sugar: 14 g

Cinnaminis

No rise, no wait—these amazing little cinnamon buns can be made anytime!

INGREDIENTS | YIELDS 16

1¾ cups all-purpose flour

2 tablespoons unsalted butter, melted and cooled

⅔ cup low-fat milk

1½ teaspoons dry active yeast

¼ cup sugar

1 egg, room temperature

1 tablespoon unsalted butter, melted and cooled

¼ cup light brown sugar

1 teaspoon ground cinnamon

1½ tablespoons mascarpone cheese

3 tablespoons powdered sugar

1 teaspoon low-fat milk

1. Preheat oven to 425°F. Spray the bottom of an 8-inch square pan lightly with oil and/or line with parchment.

2. Measure flour, butter, milk, yeast, sugar, and egg into a mixing bowl and stir well to form a dough. Turn out onto a lightly floured surface and knead until smooth, adding as much as ¼ cup additional flour.

3. Roll dough out into a (roughly) 10" × 16" rectangle, keeping the long edge facing you. Brush the surface of the dough with the tablespoon of melted butter.

4. Combine the brown sugar and cinnamon in a small mixing bowl and sprinkle evenly over the surface of the dough.

5. Starting at the long edge facing you, roll the dough away from you, tightly. When you get to the long edge opposite, wet the lip of the dough very lightly with water and pinch to close.

6. Cut the dough into 16 equal pieces and place the rounds (cut-side down) in the prepared pan. Place pan on middle rack in oven and bake for 15–20 minutes.

7. While cinnaminis are baking, prepare the icing. In a small bowl, beat together the mascarpone cheese, powdered sugar, and milk. Set aside.

8. Remove pan from oven and set on wire rack to cool. Cool at least 5 minutes. Drizzle icing over the cinnaminis and serve.

PER SERVING (1 CINNAMINI) | Calories: 110 | Fat: 3 g | Protein: 2 g | Sodium: 11 mg | Fiber: <1 g | Carbohydrates: 18 g | Sugar: 8 g

Perfect Crumb-Topped Coffeecake

*Classic coffeecake, reinvented! Less fat, less sugar, but all the moist flavor you love.
Bake as suggested or add fruit, chocolate chips, or citrus zest to the batter.*

INGREDIENTS | SERVES 16

¼ cup brown sugar

3 tablespoons unbleached all-purpose flour

½ teaspoon ground cinnamon

5 tablespoons unsalted butter, divided

⅔ cup sugar

½ cup low-fat vanilla yogurt

1 egg white

1 teaspoon pure vanilla extract

2 teaspoons sodium-free baking powder

½ teaspoon sodium-free baking soda

1½ cups unbleached all-purpose flour

2 tablespoons low-fat milk

Sodium-Free Baking Soda

Standard baking soda contains over 1,200 mg of sodium per teaspoon, and is not recommended for those on a DASH diet. Ener-G sodium-free baking soda substitute is an effective replacement for standard baking soda. In addition to being sodium free, it's also free of aluminum and gluten. Ener-G sodium-free baking soda substitute is sold online.

1. Preheat oven to 350°F. Lightly grease and flour an 8-inch square baking pan and set aside.

2. To make the crumb topping, mix together the brown sugar, 3 tablespoons flour, and ground cinnamon. Cut 1 tablespoon butter into the mixture until it becomes crumbly. Set aside.

3. Beat the remaining 4 tablespoons butter with the sugar. Add the yogurt, egg white, and vanilla and mix until smooth.

4. Add the baking powder and soda, then gradually add in the flour. Stir in the milk.

5. Spread batter in the prepared pan. Sprinkle the crumb topping evenly over the batter.

6. Place pan on middle rack in oven and bake for 30 minutes. Remove from oven and set on wire rack to cool briefly before cutting into slices and serving.

PER SERVING | Calories: 133 | Fat: 4 g | Protein: 2 g | Sodium: 9 mg | Fiber: <1 g | Carbohydrates: 22 g | Sugar: 11 g

CHAPTER 5

Dips, Condiments, Marinades, and More

Basil Pesto

Harvest that fragrant bounty of basil and enjoy it to its fullest. Stir a little bit into pasta or rice for a taste sensation, or use it as a spread for sandwiches, topping for pizza, and more.

INGREDIENTS | YIELDS ½ CUP

2 cups fresh basil leaves

4 cloves garlic

3 tablespoons olive oil

¼ cup pine nuts

2 tablespoons grated Parmesan cheese

¼ teaspoon freshly ground black pepper

1. Place all the ingredients into a food processor and pulse until smooth.

2. Use immediately or store in an airtight container and refrigerate until use.

PER SERVING (2 TABLESPOONS) | Calories: 166 | Fat: 17 g | Protein: 2 g | Sodium: 39 mg | Fiber: <1 g | Carbohydrates: 2 g | Sugar: <1 g

Grow Your Own

Fresh herbs are easy and inexpensive to grow in almost any living situation. A sunny windowsill or patio planter can produce enough to flavor a wide array of recipes for months to come. A few bargain pots, some soil, and seeds are all you need to get started. Whichever herbs you like best, enjoy them conveniently and at their freshest by growing your own.

Cilantro Peanut Pesto

A flavorful change from standard basil pesto, this zesty Asian-inspired sauce is great on grains, pasta, and more.

INGREDIENTS | YIELDS ½ CUP

½ cup fresh cilantro

¼ cup light coconut milk

¼ cup unsalted peanuts

4 cloves garlic

Juice and zest of 1 fresh lime

1. Place all the ingredients into a food processor and pulse until smooth.

2. Use immediately or store in an airtight container and refrigerate until use.

PER SERVING | Calories: 79 | Fat: 5 g | Protein: 2 g | Sodium: 5 mg | Fiber: 1 g | Carbohydrates: 6 g | Sugar: 2 g

Fat-Free Black Bean Dip

Completely guilt free and so good! A chorus line of black beans, cilantro, and garlic with a zippy lime high kick. Serve with fresh vegetables, unsalted tortilla chips, or as a filling or topping for burritos.

INGREDIENTS | YIELDS 1½ CUPS

1 (15-ounce) can no-salt-added black beans

¼ cup fresh cilantro

2 cloves garlic

Juice of 1 fresh lime

1½ teaspoons ground cumin

½ teaspoon ground coriander

⅛ teaspoon ground cayenne

1. Drain black beans and rinse well.

2. Place all the ingredients in a food processor and pulse until smooth.

3. Serve immediately or cover and refrigerate until serving.

PER SERVING (2 TABLESPOONS) | Calories: 49 | Fat: <1 g | Protein: 3 g | Sodium: 1 mg | Fiber: 3 g | Carbohydrates: 9 g | Sugar: 0 g

Squeeze Your Citrus

To get the most out of citrus fruit, give it a squeeze! Before juicing, roll citrus on the counter, pressing down firmly with your hands. The pressure will allow more of the juice to be extracted and it'll make your hands smell great, too! Another tip: When citrus gets old, it often dries out inside. Microwave older fruit for 15 seconds to get the most juice from your squeeze.

Sour Cream and Onion Dip

This rich, creamy, and guilt-free alternative to commercial dips makes a terrific topping for baked potatoes, stir-in for scrambled eggs, and partner for fresh-cut veggies.

INGREDIENTS | YIELDS 1 CUP (16 TABLESPOON SERVINGS)

1 medium onion, diced

1 cup nonfat sour cream

1 teaspoon all-purpose salt-free seasoning

¼ teaspoon garlic powder

1. Sauté the onion over medium heat until soft and brown, roughly 3–5 minutes.

2. Place the remaining ingredients into a small mixing bowl. Add sautéed onion and stir well to combine.

3. Cover and refrigerate until serving.

PER SERVING (1 TABLESPOON) | Calories: 23 | Fat: 0 g | Protein: 1 g | Sodium: 42 mg | Fiber: 0 g | Carbohydrates: 4 g | Sugar: 0 g

Holy Guacamole

Vibrant in color and flavor, this simple dip makes any meal more special. Serve with everything from chips to tacos to rice and beans. Guacamole is best consumed fresh, so serve the same day.

INGREDIENTS | YIELDS 1 CUP

1 ripe avocado

1 small ripe tomato, chopped

Juice of 1 fresh lime

1 or 2 cloves garlic, minced

1 tablespoon chopped fresh cilantro

½ teaspoon ground cumin

Pinch ground cayenne pepper

1. Peel, pit, and dice the avocado. Place diced avocado in a deep bowl and mash with a fork, as smoothly or coarsely as desired.

2. Add remaining ingredients and mix well.

3. Serve immediately or cover and chill before serving.

PER SERVING (2 TABLESPOONS) | Calories: 45 | Fat: 3 g | Protein: 0 g | Sodium: 3 mg | Fiber: 2 g | Carbohydrates: 3 g | Sugar: 0 g

Avocado Facts

Avocados are native to South and Central America and are actually a fruit, not a vegetable. Ripe avocados have a smooth, leathery skin that when ripe yields gently to pressure. The easiest way to prepare a ripe avocado is to cut lengthwise through the fruit to the core, gently break open, remove pit, and peel away skin. Avocados are high in vitamins B_6, C, E, and K, and have been shown to protect against prostate cancer.

Roasted Red Pepper Hummus

Flavored by succulent roasted pepper, this colorful dip is great with chips or veggies, and also makes a wonderful low-sodium sandwich spread.

INGREDIENTS | YIELDS 1½ CUPS

1 (15-ounce) can no-salt-added garbanzo beans

⅓ cup Roasted Red Peppers (see Chapter 15)

2 cloves garlic

2 tablespoons freshly squeezed lemon juice

2 tablespoons sesame tahini

1. Drain garbanzo beans and rinse well.

2. Place all the ingredients in a food processor and pulse until smooth.

3. Serve immediately or cover and refrigerate until serving.

PER SERVING (2 TABLESPOONS) | Calories: 79 | Fat: 2 g | Protein: 3 g | Sodium: 6 mg | Fiber: 3 g | Carbohydrates: 12 g | Sugar: 2 g

Garlic Lovers Hummus

The ultimate vegetarian dip and sandwich filling. This version calls for tahini, a smooth sesame butter sold in many supermarkets and natural food stores. If you can't find it, try substituting low-sodium vegetable broth. For a milder flavor, reduce the amount of garlic.

INGREDIENTS | YIELDS 1½ CUPS

1 (15-ounce) can no-salt-added garbanzo beans
3 tablespoons sesame tahini
3 tablespoons freshly squeezed lemon juice
2 tablespoons olive oil
4 cloves garlic

1. Drain garbanzo beans and rinse well.

2. Place all the ingredients in a food processor and pulse until smooth.

3. Serve immediately or cover and refrigerate until serving.

PER SERVING (2 TABLESPOONS) | Calories: 103 | Fat: 5 g | Protein: 4 g | Sodium: 7 mg | Fiber: 3 g | Carbohydrates: 11 g | Sugar: 2 g

Under Pressure

Pressure cookers make low-sodium dieting cheaper, faster, and easier. Not only do they speed up cooking time, making food preparation more convenient, but they also eliminate the need to buy often-expensive specialized no-salt-added canned goods, such as beans.

Pineapple Salsa

Fresh, ripe fruits make the best salsas, and juicy pineapple is among the best. Add an extra jalapeño or two for fire.

INGREDIENTS | YIELDS 3 CUPS

½ fresh pineapple, finely diced
1 jalapeño pepper, minced
1 small red bell pepper, diced
3 cloves garlic, minced
Juice of 1 fresh lime
¼ cup chopped fresh cilantro

1. Place all the ingredients in a bowl and stir well to combine.

2. Serve immediately or cover and refrigerate until ready to serve.

PER SERVING (2 TABLESPOONS) | Calories: 14 | Fat: 0 g | Protein: 0 g | Sodium: 1 mg | Fiber: 0 g | Carbohydrates: 4 g | Sugar: 2 g

Orange Cranberry Sauce

This thick relish makes a superb low-sodium sandwich topping, addition to breakfast, or garnish for roasted meat.

INGREDIENTS | YIELDS 2 CUPS

3 cups fresh whole cranberries
1 clementine
1 cup freshly squeezed orange juice
1 cup sugar

1. Wash the cranberries well and set aside.

2. Peel, segment, and coarsely chop the clementine. Set aside.

3. Place the juice and sugar into a small stockpot and stir to combine. Bring to a boil over high heat.

4. Add the cranberries and clementine, reduce heat to medium, and simmer for 10 minutes.

5. Remove from heat and cover. Allow to cool to room temperature before serving.

PER SERVING (2 TABLESPOONS) | Calories: 66 | Fat: 0 g | Protein: 0 g | Sodium: 1 mg | Fiber: 1 g | Carbohydrates: 17 g | Sugar: 15 g

Peach Salsa

Save this salsa for the peak of summer, when ripe peaches are in endless supply. You'll want to keep enjoying it, and enjoying it, over and again.

INGREDIENTS | YIELDS 3 CUPS

3 ripe peaches, peeled and diced
1 ripe tomato, diced
1 small bell pepper, diced
1 jalapeño pepper, minced
2 cloves garlic, minced
2 tablespoons chopped fresh cilantro
1 tablespoon apple cider vinegar
1½ teaspoons unsweetened apple juice
1½ teaspoons honey
1 teaspoon ground cumin
½ teaspoon ground coriander

1. Place all the ingredients in a bowl and stir well to combine.

2. Serve immediately or cover and refrigerate until ready to serve.

PER SERVING | Calories: 12 | Fat: 0 g | Protein: 0 g | Sodium: 1 mg | Fiber: <1 g | Carbohydrates: 3 g | Sugar: 2 g

Chunky Unsweetened Applesauce

This salt-free natural applesauce is delicious on its own, spooned over latkes or pancakes, or served as a condiment with grilled meat.

INGREDIENTS | YIELDS 5 CUPS

10 medium apples, any variety
1 cup unsweetened apple juice

Cut the Fat!

When looking to minimize oil in baked goods, try substituting unsweetened applesauce, mashed banana, or puréed prunes for all or part of the fat. When sautéing, coat the bottom of pans with water or fat-free low-sodium broth. Little steps like this add up, and will keep you slimmer and healthier.

1. Peel, core, and dice the apples.

2. Place diced apples into a large pot, add the apple juice, and bring to a boil over medium-high heat.

3. Reduce heat to low and simmer uncovered, stirring frequently. Cook until apples are tender and falling apart, roughly 20–30 minutes.

4. Remove from heat and mash coarsely using a potato masher.

5. Spoon into clean lidded jars and refrigerate until ready to serve.

PER SERVING (½ CUP) | Calories: 58 | Fat: 0 g | Protein: 0 g | Sodium: 1 mg | Fiber: 1 g | Carbohydrates: 15 g | Sugar: 12 g

Spicy Lime, Cilantro, and Garlic Marinade

The most amazing citrusy, garlicky, spicy Southwestern taste imaginable. Thanks to Tammy and Sarita for sharing!

INGREDIENTS | YIELDS 1 CUP

2 teaspoons olive oil
½ cup finely chopped fresh cilantro
4 cloves garlic, minced
1 tablespoon dried red pepper flakes
¼ cup freshly squeezed lime juice (juice of 2 limes)

1. Measure the olive oil into a mixing bowl.

2. Add the chopped cilantro, garlic, and red pepper flakes, then stir to combine.

3. Add the lime juice and mix well.

4. Place meat or tofu in the marinade and toss gently to coat. Refrigerate until ready to cook.

PER SERVING (1 CUP) | Calories: 112 | Fat: 9 g | Protein: 1 g | Sodium: 3 mg | Fiber: 0 g | Carbohydrates: 9 g | Sugar: 1 g

Mango Salsa

Ripe mangoes, garlic, lime, and cilantro flavor one of the most mouth-wateringly tasty salsas ever.

INGREDIENTS | YIELDS 2 CUPS

1 ripe mango, peeled and diced

1 small red bell pepper, chopped

2 cloves garlic, minced

1 jalapeño pepper, minced

Juice of 1 fresh lime

2 tablespoons chopped fresh cilantro

1 tablespoon apple cider vinegar

1 teaspoon agave nectar

1 teaspoon ground cumin

1. Place all the ingredients in a bowl and stir well to combine.

2. Serve immediately or cover and refrigerate until ready to serve.

PER SERVING (2 TABLESPOONS) | Calories: 16 | Fat: 0 g | Protein: 0 g | Sodium: 1 mg | Fiber: 0 g | Carbohydrates: 4 g | Sugar: 3 g

Strawberry Salsa

A truly stellar salsa made from fresh strawberries. The cinnamon adds depth to the triumvirate of spicy, sweet, and savory flavors.

INGREDIENTS | YIELDS 2 CUPS

2 cups chopped fresh strawberries

1 small yellow or orange bell pepper. chopped

1 jalapeño pepper, minced

2 cloves garlic, minced

2 tablespoons chopped fresh cilantro

Juice of 1 fresh lemon

2 teaspoons agave nectar

1 teaspoon minced fresh ginger

½ teaspoon ground cinnamon

½ teaspoon ground cumin

1. Place all the ingredients in a bowl and stir well to combine.

2. Serve immediately or cover and refrigerate until ready to serve.

PER SERVING (2 TABLESPOONS) | Calories: 12 | Fat: 0 g | Protein: 0 g | Sodium: 1 mg | Fiber: <1 g | Carbohydrates: 3 g | Sugar: 2 g

Roasted Tomato Salsa

A delicious, flavorful salsa with roasted tomato, pepper, and onion. This recipe is fairly mild; to increase the heat, leave the jalapeño seeds in or add additional hot peppers.

INGREDIENTS | YIELDS 2 CUPS

5 medium tomatoes
1 medium green bell pepper
1 medium onion
3 cloves garlic, minced
1 jalapeño pepper, minced
1 tablespoon chopped fresh cilantro
3 tablespoons apple cider vinegar
1 teaspoon ground cumin
⅛ teaspoon liquid smoke

1. Preheat oven to 450°F. Spray a baking sheet lightly with oil.

2. Slice the tomatoes in half and place cut-side down on baking sheet. Slice the bell pepper in half, remove core and seeds, and place cut-side down on baking sheet. Trim onion, slice in half, and place cut-side down on baking sheet. Place pan on middle rack in oven and roast for 15 minutes.

3. Remove baking sheet from oven and let rest until cool enough to touch. Gently peel skins from tomatoes and pepper. Lift tomatoes from pan (they will be very soft) and gently squeeze out and discard seeds. Transfer tomato pulp to a mixing bowl.

4. Chop the roasted pepper and onion and add to bowl.

5. Add the remaining ingredients to the bowl and stir well to combine.

6. Serve immediately or cover and refrigerate until ready to serve.

PER SERVING (2 TABLESPOONS) | Calories: 11 | Fat: 0 g | Protein: 0 g | Sodium: 3 mg | Fiber: <1 g | Carbohydrates: 2 g | Sugar: 1 g

Faux Soy Sauce

Meet soy sauce's tasty cousin, Faux. Partnered with other Asian ingredients, you'll never know the difference. Adapted from Dick Logue's Soy Sauce Substitute.

INGREDIENTS | YIELDS ⅔ CUP

¼ cup molasses

3 tablespoons unflavored rice wine vinegar

1 tablespoon water

1 teaspoon sodium-free beef bouillon granules

½ teaspoon freshly ground black pepper

1. Place all the ingredients into a small saucepan or microwave-safe bowl and heat on low to combine, roughly 1 minute.

2. Use immediately or store in an airtight container and refrigerate until ready to use.

PER SERVING (1 TABLESPOON) | Calories: 25 | Fat: 0 g | Protein: 0 g | Sodium: 3 mg | Fiber: 0 g | Carbohydrates: 6 g | Sugar: 4 g

Molasses Alert!

When making Faux Soy Sauce and other dishes, look for the lowest-sodium molasses you can find. Grandma's Original Unsulphured Molasses and Crosby's Fancy Molasses are both very low in sodium. If you can't locate either, check labels carefully before purchase. Some molasses brands contain high levels of sodium; it's better to be safe than sorry.

Asian-Inspired Low-Sodium Marinade

Adapted from Cooking Light, this low-sodium marinade has subtle nuances of garlic and ginger, 5-spice powder, and the sweet tang of rice wine vinegar.

INGREDIENTS | YIELDS ½ CUP

3 tablespoons Faux Soy Sauce (see previous)

1½ tablespoons honey

1 tablespoon unflavored rice wine vinegar

1½ teaspoons canola oil

2 garlic cloves, minced

1½ tablespoons grated fresh ginger

¼ teaspoon 5-spice powder

Freshly ground black pepper, to taste

1. Combine all the ingredients in a large, zip-top plastic bag. Add choice of meat, tofu, or other protein and seal bag tightly.

2. Shake and/or invert several times to coat contents completely.

3. Refrigerate at least 2 hours, turning occasionally. Remove contents and prepare as desired.

PER SERVING (1 TABLESPOON) | Calories: 32 | Fat: 1 g | Protein: 0 g | Sodium: 2 mg | Fiber: 0 g | Carbohydrates: 6 g | Sugar: 5 g

Salt-Free Mayonnaise

Adapted from Southern Living Magazine, *this light and creamy mayonnaise uses liquid egg substitute, eliminating cholesterol and the risk of salmonella.*

INGREDIENTS | YIELDS 1 CUP

¼ cup liquid egg substitute (e.g., Egg Beaters)

2½ tablespoons distilled white vinegar

½ teaspoon white pepper

⅛ teaspoon garlic powder

⅛ teaspoon dry ground mustard

Pinch ground cayenne pepper

⅔ cup canola oil

Liquid Egg Substitutes

Sold in cartons beside the eggs, liquid egg substitutes such as Egg Beaters are a great way of enjoying the flavor of whole eggs without the fat and cholesterol. Substitute ¼ cup of liquid egg substitute for each egg in most recipes without a discernable difference in taste or texture. Liquid egg substitutes can be frozen as well, making them both healthy and convenient.

1. Place all of the ingredients except the oil into a food processor and pulse until smooth. Scrape down sides.

2. With food processor running, add the oil in a slow and steady stream until thickened.

3. Store mayonnaise in a clean lidded jar and refrigerate when not in use.

PER SERVING (1 TABLESPOON) | Calories: 84 | Fat: 9 g | Protein: 0 g | Sodium: 7 mg | Fiber: 0 g | Carbohydrates: 0 g | Sugar: 0 g

Spicy, Sweet, and Tangy Barbecue Sauce

Salt free, fat free, and absolutely amazing! An authentic-tasting BBQ sauce for all your grilling, basting, and dipping needs.

INGREDIENTS | YIELDS 2 CUPS

2 (8-ounce) cans no-salt-added tomato sauce

3 tablespoons apple cider vinegar

2 tablespoons molasses

1 tablespoon honey

1 teaspoon liquid smoke

2 teaspoons onion powder

1½ teaspoons ground cumin

1 teaspoon ground sweet paprika

½ teaspoon garlic powder

½ teaspoon freshly ground black pepper

⅛ teaspoon ground cayenne pepper

1. Combine ingredients in a saucepan and simmer over medium-low heat for 10 minutes.

2. Remove from heat and pour into a clean lidded jar. Refrigerate until ready to use.

PER SERVING (2 TABLESPOONS) | Calories: 24 | Fat: 0 g | Protein: 0 g | Sodium: 4 mg | Fiber: 0 g | Carbohydrates: 5 g | Sugar: 4 g

Salt-Free Dijon Mustard

Spicy and sophisticated, this mustard brings the best out of almost anything from grilled meat to sandwiches and salad dressings.

INGREDIENTS | YIELDS ½ CUP

⅓ cup dry ground mustard

2 tablespoons white wine

½ cup white distilled vinegar

½ cup water

1 teaspoon garlic powder

1. Place all the ingredients into a small saucepan and stir well to combine.

2. Bring to a boil over medium heat. Once boiling, lower heat to medium-low and simmer, stirring frequently, until thickened, 20–25 minutes.

3. Pour mustard into a clean lidded jar and refrigerate until ready to use.

PER SERVING (1 TABLESPOON) | Calories: 21 | Fat: 0 g | Protein: 0 g | Sodium: 1 mg | Fiber: 0 g | Carbohydrates: 2 g | Sugar: 0 g

Salt-Free Ketchup

No need to purchase commercial salt-free ketchup when it's this easy to make at home. No artificial additives, preservatives, or sweeteners, and it's delicious!

INGREDIENTS | YIELDS 3 CUPS (48 TABLESPOON SERVINGS)

3 (8-ounce) cans no-salt-added tomato sauce

5 tablespoons no-salt-added tomato paste

3 tablespoons distilled white vinegar

5 teaspoons sugar

¼ teaspoon garlic powder

¼ teaspoon onion powder

⅛ teaspoon dry ground mustard

⅛ teaspoon ground cinnamon

⅛ teaspoon ground cumin

1. Measure all the ingredients into a 3-quart saucepan and stir until completely smooth.

2. Place pan over medium heat. As soon as mixture begins to bubble, reduce heat to low and simmer for 10 minutes.

3. Remove from heat and pour ketchup into a clean lidded jar. Refrigerate when not using.

PER SERVING (1 TABLESPOON) | Calories: 9 | Fat: 0 g | Protein: 0 g | Sodium: 3 mg | Fiber: 0 g | Carbohydrates: 2 g | Sugar: 1 g

Tips to Reduce Dietary Sodium

Seek out products that are labeled "salt free" or "no salt added." Canned goods such as tomatoes, vegetables, and beans all come in salt-free varieties. And don't forget the condiments! Salt-free versions of ketchup, mustard, even pickles, are all available in supermarkets and online. Salt-free products will save you hundreds of mg of sodium per serving.

Homemade Honey Mustard

This delicious salt-free mustard takes only 5 minutes to prepare and yields a sweet and zingy mustard as good as any gourmet brand. Many thanks to Judi for sharing!

INGREDIENTS | YIELDS ¾ CUP

½ cup dry mustard
½ cup distilled white vinegar
¼ cup honey
1 tablespoon canola oil
¼ teaspoon ground allspice
¼ teaspoon garlic powder
¼ teaspoon freshly ground black pepper

Chef's Note

Homemade mustard will thicken significantly when refrigerated, so don't be concerned if it appears somewhat loose right after the cooking time has ended. Homemade mustard will keep for weeks in the refrigerator. Store it in a clean lidded jar, labeled with the date, if possible.

1. Combine all the ingredients in a small saucepan. Place over medium-high heat and stir constantly until boiling.

2. Once boiling, reduce heat to medium-low. Continue boiling until mustard begins to thicken, roughly 5 minutes.

3. Pour into a clean lidded jar and refrigerate until ready to use. Mustard will thicken significantly in the refrigerator.

PER SERVING (1 TABLESPOON) | Calories: 44 | Fat: 1 g | Protein: 0 g | Sodium: 0 mg | Fiber: 0 g | Carbohydrates: 6 g | Sugar: 5 g

Low-Sodium Cocktail Sauce

Commercial cocktail sauce is high in sodium, making it a poor choice on a salt-free diet. Here's a spicy, tangy, and almost identical stand-in!

INGREDIENTS | YIELDS 1 CUP

5 tablespoons no-salt-added tomato paste
3 tablespoons apple cider vinegar
3 tablespoons molasses
2 tablespoons prepared horseradish
2 teaspoons dry ground mustard
1 clove garlic, grated

1. Place all the ingredients into a small mixing bowl and stir well to combine.

2. Chill for at least 1 hour before serving.

PER SERVING (1 TABLESPOON) | Calories: 15 | Fat: 0 g | Protein: 0 g | Sodium: 8 mg | Fiber: 0 g | Carbohydrates: 4 g | Sugar: 2 g

Instant Salt-Free Pasta Sauce

A terrific recipe for times when you run short of sauce. This recipe makes 24 ounces, equivalent to many commercial jars. All you need are canned, no-salt-added tomatoes.

INGREDIENTS | YIELDS 3 CUPS

1 (28-ounce) can no-salt-added crushed, diced, or whole tomatoes

2 teaspoons sugar

1 tablespoon onion powder

1½ teaspoons dried Italian seasoning

1 teaspoon garlic powder

½ teaspoon freshly ground black pepper

¼ teaspoon fennel seed

1. Combine all the ingredients in food processor and purée.

2. Warm in saucepan or microwave.

3. Store sauce in a clean lidded jar and refrigerate.

PER SERVING (¼ CUP) | Calories: 17 | Fat: 0 g | Protein: 0 g | Sodium: 7 mg | Fiber: 0 g | Carbohydrates: 4 g | Sugar: 2 g

Hidden Salt

Salt is one of those sneaky substances. Unless you're watching how much of it you're consuming, as in counting mg, you'd never guess how much is in most "normal" foods, like pasta sauce. Commercial pasta sauce contains on average 500 mg of sodium per serving, sometimes more. When buying pasta sauce, it's important to seek out salt-free varieties. Francesco Rinaldi's No-Salt-Added Traditional Pasta Sauce and Trader Joe's Organic No-Salt-Added Marinara Sauce are both inexpensive and very tasty.

Salt-Free Chili Seasoning

If you have difficulty finding commercial salt-free chili seasoning, make your own! It's quick, affordable, and seasonings can be adjusted to suit your taste.

NGREDIENTS | YIELDS ⅓ CUP

2 tablespoons ground cumin

1 tablespoon ground coriander

2 teaspoons dried oregano

1½ teaspoons ground sweet paprika

½ teaspoon dried red pepper flakes

½ teaspoon garlic powder

½ teaspoon onion powder

¼ teaspoon dry ground mustard

⅛ teaspoon ground cayenne pepper

1. Measure all the ingredients into a small mixing bowl and whisk well to combine.

2. Store seasoning in a small lidded jar.

PER SERVING | Calories: 0 | Fat: 0 g | Protein: 0 g | Sodium: 0 mg | Fiber: 0 g | Carbohydrates: 0 g | Sugar: 0 g

Salt-Free Italian Seasoning

A basic dried-herb blend for pasta dishes, pizza crust, and more.

INGREDIENTS | YIELDS ⅓ CUP

2 tablespoons dried basil

1 tablespoon dried oregano

2 teaspoons dried rosemary

1½ teaspoons dried thyme

1 teaspoon dried marjoram

½ teaspoon ground sage

1. Measure all the ingredients into a small mixing bowl and whisk well to combine.

2. Store seasoning in a small lidded jar.

PER SERVING | Calories: 0 | Fat: 0 g | Protein: 0 g | Sodium: 0 mg | Fiber: 0 g | Carbohydrates: 0 g | Sugar: 0 g

Preserving Dried Herbs and Spices

Many people position their spice rack close to the stove for easy access during cooking. But the proximity to heat and humidity compromises flavor and longevity. To maximize freshness, store dried herbs and spices in a cool, dark cabinet away from direct sunlight and cooking.

CHAPTER 6

Drinks

Ginger Lemonade

There's nothing so refreshing on a hot day as a glass of ice-cold lemonade.
Here, the spicy flavor and aroma of ginger adds depth, sophistication, and kick.

INGREDIENTS | SERVES 4

¼ cup minced fresh ginger
Minced zest of 1 fresh lemon
1 cup freshly squeezed lemon juice
3 cups water
5 tablespoons sugar

1. Place the minced ginger and lemon zest into a small pitcher. Add the lemon juice, water, and sugar, and stir well to combine.

2. Place pitcher in refrigerator and allow mixture to steep at least 4 hours for flavors to fully develop.

3. When ready to serve, fill 4 tall glasses with ice, pour lemonade over the ice, and serve.

PER SERVING | Calories: 75 | Fat: 0 g | Protein: 0 g | Sodium: 8 mg | Fiber: 0 g | Carbohydrates: 21 g | Sugar: 17 g

Cranberry Limeade

Cranberry juice and lime are a match made in heaven.
Sweet, tart, and tangy, it's best served ice cold.

INGREDIENTS | SERVES 6

1 cup freshly squeezed lime juice
Grated zest of 1 fresh lime
3 cups water
1 cup cranberry juice (100% juice blend)
¼ cup sugar

1. Measure all the ingredients into a large pitcher and stir well to combine.

2. Serve immediately or refrigerate until ready to serve.

PER SERVING | Calories: 62 | Fat: 0 g | Protein: 0 g | Sodium: 6 mg | Fiber: 0 g | Carbohydrates: 17 g | Sugar: 14 g

Cranberry Facts

Cranberries contain numerous antioxidants, high levels of vitamin C, and have even been reported to inhibit cancer. But perhaps what they're best known for is their ability to protect against urinary tract infections. A substance within the cranberry is thought to prevent bacteria from adhering to the bladder wall, thus preventing attack.

Ruby Red Grapefruit Spritzers

*An irresistibly rosy hue and mint freshness make these cocktails
a satisfying alternative to champagne.*

INGREDIENTS | SERVES 4

1 teaspoon chopped fresh mint
¾ cup ruby red grapefruit juice
12 ounces unflavored seltzer water

1. Divide mint evenly among 4 champagne flutes.

2. Add an equal amount of grapefruit juice to each glass, then top with seltzer.

3. Serve immediately.

PER SERVING | Calories: 18 | Fat: 0 g | Protein: 0 g | Sodium: 0 mg | Fiber: 0 g | Carbohydrates: 4 g | Sugar: 3 g

Lemon Iced Tea

*Use standard black tea for a traditional flavor or get creative with different herbal blends.
Agave nectar melds fluidly with the tea; substitute honey or another sweetener if you prefer.*

INGREDIENTS | SERVES 6

6 tea bags
6 cups water
Juice of 1–2 fresh lemons
4 tablespoons agave nectar

Tea Facts

Tea has been enjoyed for thousands of years and is associated not only with hydration and refreshment but with ritual. Tea leaves contain hundreds of antioxidants said to reduce the risk of cancer and other diseases. Whether enjoyed hot or cold, in beverage form or added to food, caffeinated or not, tea is something to be savored and cherished.

1. Place tea bags into a large heatproof pitcher.

2. Measure water into a kettle or saucepan and place over high heat. Once water begins to steam but not boil, remove from heat and pour into pitcher.

3. Let tea steep 3–5 minutes, depending upon taste. Remove tea bags from pitcher and discard. Add lemon juice and agave nectar and stir well to combine.

4. Let tea cool at room temperature or place pitcher in refrigerator and chill before serving.

PER SERVING | Calories: 45 | Fat: 0 g | Protein: 0 g | Sodium: 9 mg | Fiber: 0 g | Carbohydrates: 11 g | Sugar: 10 g

Green Mango Smoothies

Tender baby spinach gives these smoothies their bright color and nutrient boost. The sweet and fruity flavor hides the spinach well; close your eyes and you'd never guess it's in there!

INGREDIENTS | SERVES 4

1 cup baby spinach
1 ripe kiwi fruit
1 ripe banana
1 cup mango juice
½ cup low-fat vanilla yogurt

1. Place spinach into a blender or food processor and purée.

2. Add the kiwi and banana and purée again.

3. Add remaining ingredients and pulse until smooth and creamy.

4. Serve immediately.

PER SERVING | Calories: 98 | Fat: 0 g | Protein: 2 g | Sodium: 20 mg | Fiber: 2 g | Carbohydrates: 20 g | Sugar: 13 g

Peanut Butter Banana Smoothies

A protein- and potassium-packed power breakfast! Choose vanilla nondairy milk if you prefer a little more sweetness, plain if not.

INGREDIENTS | SERVES 2

2 tablespoons no-salt-added peanut butter
2 ripe bananas
1 cup nondairy milk

Go Bananas for Bananas

Whether eaten out of hand or puréed into a smoothie, bananas are one of the best on-the-go breakfasts possible. Loaded with vitamins B6 and C, fiber, and potassium, and packaged in a perfect portable container, bananas are one of the healthiest, fat-free snacks ever.

1. Place the peanut butter and bananas into a blender or food processor and purée, scraping down sides as necessary.

2. Add the nondairy milk and pulse until smooth and creamy.

3. Serve immediately.

PER SERVING | Calories: 238 | Fat: 10 g | Protein: 8 g | Sodium: 48 mg | Fiber: 4 g | Carbohydrates: 32 g | Sugar: 16 g

Orange Creamsicle Smoothies

A healthy vegan shake with a deliciously decadent taste.
These creamsicle smoothies are just like the frozen treats, but better.

INGREDIENTS | SERVES 2

1 large navel orange
1 cup vanilla nondairy milk

1. Peel orange, removing as much of the white pith as possible.

2. Segment orange and purée in blender or food processor. Add nondairy milk and pulse until smooth.

3. Serve immediately.

PER SERVING | Calories: 84 | Fat: 2 g | Protein: 3 g | Sodium: 57 mg | Fiber: 2 g | Carbohydrates: 14 g | Sugar: 10 g

Blueberry Pomegranate Smoothies

The ultimate in antioxidants! These powerfully delicious smoothies
have a vivid purple color and creamy sweetness.

INGREDIENTS | SERVES 3

1 cup pomegranate juice (e.g., Pom)
1 cup low-fat vanilla yogurt
⅔ cup fresh blueberries

1. Place all the ingredients into a blender or food processor and pulse until smooth and creamy.

2. Serve immediately.

PER SERVING | Calories: 116 | Fat: 1 g | Protein: 3 g | Sodium: 43 mg | Fiber: 1 g | Carbohydrates: 16 g | Sugar: 14 g

Pomegranate Facts

Pomegranates are native to Iran, and are eaten widely throughout the Middle East and beyond. The fruit is a vivid red color, inside and out, and is filled with tiny juicy seeds. For those who find the fruit difficult and tedious to eat, pomegranate juice provides all the benefits, save for the fiber. Pomegranates are a good source of folate, potassium, vitamin K, and antioxidants.

Pumpkin Coconut Smoothies

*Thick, creamy, and absolutely delicious, these pumpkin smoothies
are a great alternative to the high-fat frozen treats sold each fall.*

INGREDIENTS | SERVES 3

½ cup pumpkin purée
1 cup light coconut milk
½ cup low-fat vanilla yogurt
1 tablespoon agave nectar

1. Measure all ingredients into a blender or food processor and pulse until smooth.

2. Serve immediately.

PER SERVING | Calories: 121 | Fat: 6 g | Protein: 2 g | Sodium: 36 mg | Fiber: 1 g | Carbohydrates: 10 g | Sugar: 8 g

Chocolate-Covered Banana Milkshakes

*Decadent taste with zero guilt! These low-fat shakes are a healthy and
satisfying alternative to traditional ice cream parlor fare.*

INGREDIENTS | SERVES 2

1 ripe banana
1 cup vanilla nonfat frozen yogurt
1 tablespoon unsweetened cocoa powder
1 cup low-fat milk

1. Place banana into a blender or food processor and purée.

2. Add remaining ingredients and pulse until smooth.

3. Serve immediately.

PER SERVING | Calories: 209 | Fat: 2 g | Protein: 9 g | Sodium: 124 mg | Fiber: 2 g | Carbohydrates: 42 g | Sugar: 32 g

Blenders Versus Food Processors

Can't decide which appliance to invest in? Think about long-term use. For drinks, a blender may be the best choice. But if you're looking to purée and chop as well as blend, a food processor may be a better option. Also consider how often you will be using the appliance. For light use, an inexpensive model works well. For heavy use, invest in a large-capacity appliance with a strong motor and warranty. Do research and read reviews before deciding.

Maple Mocha Frappe

A creamy concoction of coffee, cocoa, and milk, sweetened with a touch of maple syrup. Perfect for breakfast or as an anytime pick-me-up. The stronger the coffee, the more flavor it lends to the drink.

INGREDIENTS | SERVES 4

1 small ripe banana
½ cup brewed coffee
½ cup low-fat milk
1 cup low-fat yogurt
1 tablespoon unsweetened cocoa powder
2 tablespoons pure maple syrup

1. Place the banana in a blender or food processor and purée.

2. Add the remaining ingredients and pulse until smooth and creamy.

3. Serve immediately.

PER SERVING | Calories: 103 | Fat: 1 g | Protein: 3 g | Sodium: 58 mg | Fiber: 1 g | Carbohydrates: 19 g | Sugar: 15 g

Piña Colada Smoothies

In these nonalcoholic coladas, coconut water adds the same great flavor of coconut milk without the fat. Substitute nondairy yogurt for a vegan version.

INGREDIENTS | SERVES 4

1¾ cups diced fresh pineapple
1 cup low-fat vanilla yogurt
½ cup coconut water with pulp

1. Place pineapple in food processor and purée.

2. Add remaining ingredients and pulse until smooth. Serve immediately.

PER SERVING | Calories: 84 | Fat: 1 g | Protein: 2 g | Sodium: 59 mg | Fiber: 1 g | Carbohydrates: 11 g | Sugar: 8 g

Ingredient Alert

Coconut water is sold in cans and disposable juice boxes, often in the international aisle of grocery stores. Coconut water has the same great flavor of fresh coconut, while being low in fat. Drink cold coconut water as pure refreshment, freeze as ice cubes to subtly flavor cocktails, or add to recipes for a coconut nuance.

Fat-Free Mango Milkshakes

Thick, creamy, and absolutely delicious.
If you love mango, here's your new best friend.

INGREDIENTS | SERVES 2

1 ripe mango
1 cup vanilla nonfat frozen yogurt
1 cup mango juice

1. Peel mango and cut into cubes.

2. Place into a blender or food processor and purée.

3. Add remaining ingredients and pulse until smooth.

4. Serve immediately.

PER SERVING | Calories: 239 | Fat: 0 g | Protein: 4 g |
Sodium: 72 mg | Fiber: 2 g | Carbohydrates: 56 g | Sugar: 49 g

Orange Spiced Apple Cider

There's nothing so soothing as a warm kitchen filled with the smells of apple,
cinnamon, and cloves. This spiced cider hugs like a blanket, filling you with sweetness.
Adapted from Williams-Sonoma Thanksgiving Entertaining.

INGREDIENTS | SERVES 4

1 small orange or tangerine
12 whole cloves
1 quart apple cider
4 cinnamon sticks
1 star anise pod

What Is Star Anise?

Small, brown, star-shaped seed pods, star anise come from a tree native to China. The pods have an anise or black licorice flavor, and are used in many types of cooking. The ground pods are one of the spices that goes into 5-spice powder. Try adding a star anise to a pot of your favorite tea or simmer in a stovetop potpourri.

1. Stud the orange with the cloves, pressing each in firmly to secure.

2. Place the orange in a pot and add the cider.

3. Add the cinnamon sticks and star anise.

4. Place pot over low heat. Bring contents to a simmer and keep warm over low heat until serving.

5. To serve, ladle into mugs and garnish each with a cinnamon stick.

PER SERVING | Calories: 120 | Fat: 0 g | Protein: 0 g |
Sodium: 0 mg | Fiber: 0 g | Carbohydrates: 28 g | Sugar: 26 g

Cherry Slushies

A semifrozen concoction of crystallized juice and fruit,
these slushies are pure refreshment.

INGREDIENTS | SERVES 4

1½ cups fresh pitted cherries, coarsely chopped

4 cups 100% fruit juice (your choice)

Fruit, Juice, and a Freezer

Healthy frozen treats are a terrific way to refresh body and mind. Freeze juice solid, scrape like a granita, and you've made delicious water ice. Fill plastic popsicle molds with juice, drop in fruit, and freeze for fabulous ice pops. Or use a simple ice tray, embellishing cubes with citrus zest, fresh herbs, or berries.

1. Place the cherries in an 8-inch square baking pan.

2. Pour in juice and cover tightly with plastic wrap. Carefully place in freezer for roughly 3 hours.

3. Remove from freezer and scrape/ladle into 4 glasses. Serve immediately.

PER SERVING | Calories: 140 | Fat: 0 g | Protein: 0 g | Sodium: 11 mg | Fiber: 1 g | Carbohydrates: 34 g | Sugar: 29 g

Christy's Cocktails

Slightly syrupy with the pungent taste of anise, Sambuca is an Italian liqueur people seem to either love or hate. Combined with root beer, it's transformed into a deliciously exotic cocktail.

INGREDIENTS | SERVES 2

Ice, as needed
2 ounces Sambuca
12 ounces root beer

1. Fill 2 glasses with ice.

2. Pour 1 ounce of Sambuca into each glass.

3. Divide the root beer evenly between the 2 glasses. Serve immediately.

PER SERVING | Calories: 170 | Fat: 0 g | Protein: 0 g | Sodium: 22 mg | Fiber: 0 g | Carbohydrates: 25 g | Sugar: 18 g

Donno's Mojitos

Fresh and invigorating, these Cuban cocktails will leave you begging for more. A nonalcoholic version, or Nojito, can be made without the rum. Many thanks to Donno for the wonderful recipe!

INGREDIENTS | SERVES 2

8 fresh mint leaves
Juice of 1 fresh lime
2 tablespoons turbinado sugar (e.g., Sugar in the Raw)
Ice, as needed
2 ounces white rum
12 ounces unflavored seltzer water

Different Types of Sugar

Cane sugar comes in many different varieties, the three standard types being white granulated sugar, brown sugar, and powdered or confectioners' sugar. But there are other alternatives. Evaporated cane juice, also called raw or turbinado sugar, is a natural, unrefined product that can be substituted one-for-one for granulated sugar. Demerara sugar is similar to raw sugar, but with a larger, coarser grain. It's often sprinkled on muffins or scones before baking.

1. Divide the mint leaves equally between 2 glasses. Using a wooden spoon, rub the leaves all over the insides of the glasses.

2. Divide the lime juice and sugar evenly between the 2 glasses. Use the spoon to agitate the contents, dissolving the sugar and thoroughly combining the ingredients.

3. Fill both glasses to the top with ice. Divide the rum evenly between the 2 glasses, pouring the rum over the ice.

4. Fill glasses with seltzer and garnish with additional mint leaves and/or lime wedges, if desired. Serve immediately.

PER SERVING | Calories: 117 | Fat: 0 g | Protein: 0 g | Sodium: 36 mg | Fiber: 0 g | Carbohydrates: 14 g | Sugar: 13 g

Sangria

Delicious and refreshing, sangria is perfect for summer get-togethers.
Save your quality red wine for another time; the cheap stuff works best here.

INGREDIENTS | SERVES 12

Ice, as needed
1 (1.5 liter) bottle inexpensive, fruity red wine, chilled
1 cup triple sec
1 orange, sliced
1 lemon, sliced
1 lime, sliced
1 cup lemonade

1. Place the ice into a large pitcher or gallon-sized thermos. Pour in the wine and triple sec and stir well to combine.

2. Add in the sliced fruit and lemonade and stir gently.

3. Serve immediately or chill before serving. May be refrigerated for up to 3 days.

PER SERVING | Calories: 183 | Fat: 0 g | Protein: 0 g | Sodium: 0 mg | Fiber: 0 g | Carbohydrates: 14 g | Sugar: 10 g

Cinnamon Nutmeg Hot Chocolate

Warm mugs of steamy spiced chocolate make a sublime change from the norm.
Adapted from the American Heart Association's Around the World Cookbook.

INGREDIENTS | SERVES 4

4 cups low-fat milk
¼ cup unsweetened cocoa powder
¼ cup sugar
1 teaspoon ground cinnamon
¼ teaspoon ground nutmeg
½ teaspoon pure vanilla extract
⅛ teaspoon pure almond extract

1. Place all the ingredients into a medium saucepan and whisk well to combine.

2. Place over medium heat and simmer until the mixture is warmed through, about 5 minutes.

3. Serve immediately.

PER SERVING | Calories: 168 | Fat: 3 g | Protein: 9 g | Sodium: 108 mg | Fiber: 2 g | Carbohydrates: 28 g | Sugar: 25 g

Thin Mint Cocoa

*Heaven in cocoa form. This healthy vegan version
of the traditional treat will make mouths and tummies tingle.*

INGREDIENTS | SERVES 4

3½ cups vanilla nondairy milk
¼ cup unsweetened cocoa powder
¼ cup light brown sugar
¼ teaspoon pure peppermint extract

Peppermint Facts

Peppermint is a perennial herb, and its ability to spread and take over a garden is legendary. Its distinct taste and tingly sensation is used to flavor drinks, sweets, and salads as well as many commercial products such as toothpaste. Peppermint is said to soothe upset stomachs and aid with digestive issues as well as protect against cancer.

1. Measure nondairy milk into a saucepan and place over medium-high heat.

2. Once milk begins to steam, roughly 3–5 minutes, add cocoa and brown sugar, and whisk well to combine.

3. Remove from heat. Stir in the peppermint extract and serve immediately.

PER SERVING | Calories: 134 | Fat: 4 g | Protein: 7 g | Sodium: 83 mg | Fiber: 3 g | Carbohydrates: 20 g | Sugar: 14 g

Sweet Milky Chai Tea

*Either caffeinated or decaffeinated tea works well in this recipe.
Standard commercial black tea works wonderfully, as do herbal teas
such as peppermint. Serve over ice for a refreshing treat in hot weather.*

INGREDIENTS | SERVES 6

6 tea bags
5 cups water
1 cup low-fat milk
½ cup honey
1 teaspoon pure vanilla extract
¼ teaspoon ground cloves
¼ teaspoon ground ginger
⅛ teaspoon ground allspice
⅛ teaspoon ground cardamom
⅛ teaspoon ground cinnamon

1. Place all the ingredients into a saucepan and stir well to combine.

2. Heat over high until the contents begin to steam, but have not yet boiled, roughly 5 minutes. Turn off heat and let sit 1 minute.

3. Remove tea bags and ladle into a tea pot or mugs. Serve immediately.

PER SERVING | Calories: 105 | Fat: 0 g | Protein: 1 g | Sodium: 27 mg | Fiber: 0 g | Carbohydrates: 25 g | Sugar: 25 g

CHAPTER 7

Salads and Dressings

Edamame Salad with Corn and Cranberries

A delightfully chewy, crisp, and colorful salad to brighten plates and palates year round.

INGREDIENTS | SERVES 4

1¼ cups shelled edamame

¾ cup fresh or frozen corn kernels

1 small red or orange bell pepper, diced

¼ cup dried cranberries

1 shallot, finely diced

2 tablespoons red wine vinegar

1 tablespoon olive oil

1 teaspoon agave nectar

1 teaspoon no-salt-added prepared mustard

Freshly ground black pepper, to taste

1. Place the edamame, corn, bell pepper, cranberries, and shallot in a mixing bowl and stir to combine.

2. Measure the vinegar, oil, agave nectar, and mustard into a small mixing bowl and whisk well.

3. Pour the dressing over the salad and toss to coat. Season with freshly ground black pepper, to taste.

4. Serve immediately or cover and refrigerate until ready to serve.

PER SERVING | Calories: 149 | Fat: 5 g | Protein: 5 g | Sodium: 5 mg | Fiber: 3 g | Carbohydrates: 22 g | Sugar: 10 g

Warm Asian Slaw

An elegant update on picnic fare. Here, bok choy stands in for classic cabbage and mayonnaise takes a hike in favor of a light sesame dressing. Modern, marvelous, and completely salt free!

INGREDIENTS | SERVES 4

1 tablespoon sesame oil

1 tablespoon peanut oil

2 sliced scallions

2 cloves garlic, minced

1 tablespoon minced fresh ginger

1 medium bok choy, chopped

2 medium carrots, shredded

1 tablespoon unflavored rice vinegar

½ teaspoon sugar

½ teaspoon ground white pepper

½ tablespoon toasted sesame seeds (optional)

1. Heat both oils in a skillet over medium. Add scallions, garlic, and ginger and cook, stirring, for 1 minute.

2. Add bok choy and carrots and sauté for 2 minutes. Remove from heat.

3. Place contents in a bowl. Stir in vinegar, sugar, and pepper. Garnish with sesame seeds, if desired.

4. Serve immediately or cover and refrigerate until ready to serve. Tastes equally great cold.

PER SERVING | Calories: 112 | Fat: 7 g | Protein: 3 g | Sodium: 72 mg | Fiber: 3 g | Carbohydrates: 9 g | Sugar: 4 g

Tangy Three-Bean Salad with Barley

A favorite recipe, with crisp green beans and the added heft of barley. If you prefer your green beans more tender, steam for a few minutes before adding to the salad. Many thanks to Janelle for sharing!

INGREDIENTS | SERVES 8

1 cup uncooked pearled barley

2¼ cups water

2 cups fresh green beans

1 (15-ounce) can no-salt-added kidney beans

1 (15-ounce) can no-salt-added garbanzo beans

1 medium red bell pepper, diced

1 small onion, finely chopped

2 tablespoons chopped fresh cilantro or parsley

⅓ cup canola oil

⅓ cup apple cider vinegar

⅓ cup pure maple syrup

Freshly ground black pepper, to taste

Bragg Apple Cider Vinegar

A wonderful low-sodium product, Bragg Apple Cider Vinegar is organic, raw, and unfiltered. The brownish, cobweb-like residue that collects on the bottom of each bottle, known as the "Mother," contains amazing health properties, similar to the live active cultures in yogurt. Use Bragg just as you would distilled apple cider vinegar, and enjoy the added nutrition it bestows. Bragg is sold in many supermarkets and natural food stores.

1. Measure the barley and water into a saucepan and bring to a boil over high heat.

2. Once boiling, reduce heat to low, cover, and simmer until water is absorbed, 25–30 minutes.

3. Remove pan from heat. Drain barley into a colander and rinse well.

4. Wash and trim the green beans, then cut into 2-inch pieces. Place beans in a mixing bowl.

5. Drain and rinse the canned beans, then add to the mixing bowl along with the bell pepper, onion, barley, and chopped cilantro or parsley. Stir well.

6. In a small mixing bowl, whisk together the oil, vinegar, and maple syrup. Pour over the salad and toss to coat. Season with freshly ground black pepper, to taste.

7. Flavors will strengthen and improve as ingredients are allowed to marinate, so this dish is best if covered and refrigerated several hours or even overnight.

PER SERVING | Calories: 367 | Fat: 11 g | Protein: 11 g | Sodium: 10 mg | Fiber: 11 g | Carbohydrates: 57 g | Sugar: 11 g

Bean Salad with Orange Vinaigrette

Three-bean salad with a citrus twist. Canned beans make this a snap to prepare; substitute 1¾ cups of each type of beans if you make them yourself.

INGREDIENTS | SERVES 6

1 (15-ounce) can no-salt-added kidney beans

1 (15-ounce) can no-salt-added garbanzo beans

1 (15-ounce) can no-salt-added pinto beans

2 shallots, chopped

1 medium carrot, shredded

1 small bell pepper, diced

1 small stalk celery, diced

¼ cup pure maple syrup

⅓ cup apple cider vinegar

2 tablespoons freshly squeezed orange juice

1 tablespoon olive oil

1 teaspoon grated orange zest

½ teaspoon freshly ground black pepper

1. Drain and rinse all the canned beans, then place in a mixing bowl.

2. Add the chopped shallot, shredded carrot, bell pepper, and celery and stir to combine.

3. Place the remaining ingredients into a small mixing bowl and whisk well. Pour the dressing over the salad and toss to coat.

4. Serve immediately or cover and refrigerate until ready to serve.

PER SERVING | Calories: 393 | Fat: 5 g | Protein: 19 g | Sodium: 70 mg | Fiber: 16 g | Carbohydrates: 69 g | Sugar: 13 g

Fresh Corn, Pepper, and Avocado Salad

The next time you make corn on the cob, set a few ears aside for this fabulous summer salad.

INGREDIENTS | SERVES 6

3 ears fresh cooked corn
1 medium red bell pepper
1 ripe avocado
1 jalapeño pepper, minced
1 scallion, thinly sliced
1 clove garlic, minced
Juice of 1 fresh lime
2 tablespoons olive oil
Freshly ground black pepper, to taste

Corn Facts

Corn is high in vitamin C, is a great source of both protein and fiber, and contains antioxidants associated with reduced risk of cardiovascular disease and hypertension. It can be eaten hot or cold, on the cob or in single kernels, and even popped. Corn grows easily in the home garden. Its sweet taste and vibrant color adds flavor, interest, and added nutrition to any meal.

1. Cut the kernels from the corn carefully, using a very sharp knife. Place in a mixing bowl.

2. Core and dice the red pepper and peel and dice the avocado. Add to the bowl, along with the jalapeño, sliced scallion (white and green parts), and minced garlic.

3. In a small bowl, whisk together the lime juice and oil. Drizzle over the salad and toss to coat. Season to taste with freshly ground black pepper.

4. Serve immediately or cover and refrigerate until ready to serve.

PER SERVING | Calories: 135 | Fat: 9 g | Protein: 2 g | Sodium: 5 mg | Fiber: 3 g | Carbohydrates: 13 g | Sugar: 2 g

Garlic Potato Salad

This toothsome concoction of potatoes, scallion, and garlic is hefty enough to fill, yet light enough to refresh. Enjoy with garlic scapes or clove garlic. Either way, this deliciously simple salad is a showcase of flavor. Adapted from Simply in Season.

INGREDIENTS | SERVES 6

6 medium potatoes
6 garlic scapes or 3 cloves garlic
1 cup sliced scallions
¼ cup olive oil
2 tablespoons unflavored rice vinegar
2 teaspoons chopped fresh rosemary
Freshly ground black pepper, to taste

Garlic Scapes

Long tendrils with a small bulb at one end, garlic scapes may look like something you'd simply toss into the compost, but they're a real showstopper in terms of taste. Garlic scapes are milder in flavor than their clove counterparts and can be eaten raw, minced finely, or sliced like green beans. If you've never seen or used them before, head to a summer farmers' market and pick some up.

1. Put the potatoes into a pot and add enough water to cover by 1 inch. Place over high heat and bring to a boil. Boil until fork tender but still solid, depending upon size, roughly 20–25 minutes.

2. Once cooked, remove from heat and place under cold running water. Drain and set potatoes aside to cool. Once cool enough to handle, cut into cubes.

3. Place cubed potato, garlic, and scallions into a mixing bowl and toss to combine.

4. Measure the olive oil, vinegar, and rosemary into a small mixing bowl. Add freshly ground black pepper, to taste, and whisk well to combine.

5. Pour the dressing over the salad and stir gently to coat. Cover and refrigerate a few hours before serving.

PER SERVING | Calories: 204 | Fat: 9 g | Protein: 2 g | Sodium: 6 mg | Fiber: 2 g | Carbohydrates: 28 g | Sugar: 1 g

Creamy Low-Sodium Coleslaw

Your favorite picnic fare, low-sodium style! Cabbage, carrots, and grated onion caressed in a light and creamy dressing.

INGREDIENTS | SERVES 6

½ medium head green cabbage, shredded

1 medium carrot, shredded

1 small onion, grated

⅓ cup Salt-Free Mayonnaise (see Chapter 5)

3 tablespoons sugar

3 tablespoons apple cider vinegar

½ teaspoon dry ground mustard

½ teaspoon freshly ground black pepper

1. Combine all the ingredients in a large mixing bowl and stir well.

2. Cover and refrigerate until ready to serve.

PER SERVING | Calories: 133 | Fat: 8 g | Protein: 2 g | Sodium: 32 mg | Fiber: 3 g | Carbohydrates: 13 g | Sugar: 10 g

Mayonnaise Substitute

It's hard to replace the unique taste and texture of mayonnaise, but for those watching their fat, try using nonfat sour cream instead. Before adding to a dish, measure the sour cream into a small bowl and beat in a teaspoon or two of prepared salt-free mustard. To further enhance the flavor, add a minced garlic clove and a little freshly squeezed lemon juice.

Southwestern Beet Slaw

This simple salad will make a beet lover out of you! Shredded beets are combined with carrots, scallions, garlic, cilantro, and a lime vinaigrette. The resulting salad is subtly sweet, spicy, and spectacular.

INGREDIENTS | SERVES 6

3 small–medium beets
3 scallions, sliced
2 medium carrots, shredded
¼ cup chopped fresh cilantro
2 cloves garlic
Juice of 2 fresh limes
1 teaspoon olive oil
½ teaspoon salt-free chili seasoning
¼ teaspoon freshly ground black pepper

1. Trim and peel the beets, then shred. Place into a mixing bowl.

2. Add the scallions, carrots, cilantro, and garlic and stir well to combine.

3. In a small bowl, add the lime juice, olive oil, chili seasoning, and black pepper and whisk well to combine. Pour dressing over the salad and toss well to coat.

4. Serve immediately or cover and refrigerate until ready to serve.

PER SERVING | Calories: 38 | Fat: 1 g | Protein: 1 g | Sodium: 46 mg | Fiber: 2 g | Carbohydrates: 7 g | Sugar: 4 g

Warm Kale Salad

Warm and filling, with a citrus sweetness and red pepper kick, this salad makes a great side dish or light meal.

INGREDIENTS | SERVES 4

2 teaspoons olive oil
1 small red onion, diced
2 garlic cloves, minced
1 small red bell pepper, diced
8 cups chopped kale
Juice of 1 fresh orange
1 medium carrot, shredded
¼ teaspoon ground cumin
⅛ teaspoon dried red pepper flakes
1 teaspoon grated orange zest
Freshly ground black pepper, to taste

1. Heat oil in a large skillet or sauté pan over medium. Add the onion and cook, stirring, for 2 minutes.

2. Add the garlic, bell pepper, kale, and orange juice and stir well to combine. Reduce heat to medium-low, cover, and cook for 5 minutes.

3. Remove lid, add remaining ingredients, and stir well to combine. Cover and cook for another 5 minutes.

4. Remove from heat and serve immediately.

PER SERVING | Calories: 137 | Fat: 3 g | Protein: 5 g | Sodium: 76 mg | Fiber: 4 g | Carbohydrates: 25 g | Sugar: 7 g

Tabouleh Salad

This refreshing low-sodium salad is a wonderful way to start any meal.
For a party, pair fresh veggies with tabouleh and a bowl of homemade hummus.

INGREDIENTS | SERVES 4

⅔ cup dry couscous
1 cup boiling water
1 small ripe tomato, diced
1 small green bell pepper, diced
1 shallot, finely diced
⅓ cup chopped fresh parsley
1 clove garlic, minced
Juice of 1 fresh lemon
1 tablespoon olive oil
½ teaspoon freshly ground black pepper

Parsley Facts

Parsley is an easy-growing herb that comes in two varieties: flat-leaf and curly. Too often it's dismissed as a bland plate garnish, but parsley has amazing, distinctive flavor when eaten raw. Use it to add refreshing taste and color to salads, dressings, and pastas. Parsley contains high levels of vitamins A, C, and K as well as antioxidants, and may help prevent cardiovascular disease.

1. Measure the dry couscous into a small bowl. Stir in the boiling water, cover, and set aside for 5 minutes.

2. Place the tomato, green pepper, shallot, and parsley into a salad bowl.

3. In a small mixing bowl, place the garlic, lemon juice, oil, and pepper and whisk well to combine.

4. Add the cooked couscous to the salad bowl. Pour dressing over top and stir well to combine. Serve immediately or cover and refrigerate until ready to serve.

PER SERVING | Calories: 120 | Fat: 3 g | Protein: 3 g | Sodium: 6 mg | Fiber: 1 g | Carbohydrates: 20 g | Sugar: 1 g

Tart Apple Salad with Fennel and Honey Yogurt Dressing

Crunchy and sweet with a light, refreshing finish. The fennel really makes this salad and can be used in its entirety—bulb, stalks, and fronds. Leave the peel on the apples for added nutrients and fiber.

INGREDIENTS | SERVES 6

2 tart green apples, diced

1 small bulb fennel, chopped

1½ cups seedless red grapes, halved

2 tablespoons freshly squeezed lemon juice

¼ cup low-fat vanilla yogurt

1 teaspoon honey

1. Measure all the ingredients into a mixing bowl and stir well to combine.

2. Serve immediately or cover and refrigerate until ready to serve.

PER SERVING | Calories: 70 | Fat: <1 g | Protein: 1 g | Sodium: 26 mg | Fiber: 3 g | Carbohydrates: 16 g | Sugar: 11 g

Fennel Facts

Fennel is a vegetable with a pronounced anise (black licorice) flavor and aroma. Every part of the plant is edible and can be eaten either raw or cooked. Fennel has a firm white bulb from which green celery-like stalks grow, ending in soft dill-like fronds. When it blossoms, its flowers produce small, edible, anise-flavored seeds. Fennel is high in fiber and protein, is said to alleviate stomach upset and gas, and contains antioxidants linked to preventing heart disease and cancer.

Orchid Salad

For those of you turned off by the idea of eating flowers, this dish contains none.
But when plated, there it is. An edible orchid: gorgeous and sweet, with just a hint of the exotic.

INGREDIENTS | SERVES 4

2 cups shredded red cabbage

3 tablespoons freshly squeezed orange juice

1 teaspoon balsamic vinegar

⅛ teaspoon freshly ground black pepper

2 tart green apples, sliced thinly

½ teaspoon freshly squeezed lemon juice

1 medium ripe cantaloupe

¼ cup chopped walnuts

Cantaloupe Facts

Cantaloupe, also known as muskmelon or rockmelon, has a hard, bumpy rind protecting sweet and juicy flesh. Its bright orange color is a clue to its antioxidant properties. Cantaloupe is high in beta-carotene, vitamins A and C, and has been shown to reduce the risk of high blood pressure. When selecting cantaloupe, sniff the stem end; ripe specimens will emit a sweet smell. Look for a firm exterior; soft spots may be a sign of overripe fruit.

1. Place the cabbage into a mixing bowl. Add the orange juice, vinegar, and pepper and toss well to coat. Set aside.

2. Place the apple slices in another bowl, add the lemon juice, and toss gently to coat. Set aside.

3. Slice the cantaloupe in half and remove the seeds. Slice each half into 8 wedges and remove the rind. Slice each wedge in half across the middle, so you're left with 16 triangular sections.

4. Place 2 cantaloupe sections in the middle of a plate, cut-sides together, so they look rejoined. Pull them slightly apart and then do the same with another two sections, so that you have a sort of X with an empty space in the middle.

5. Arrange a trio of fanned apple slices in each of the 4 empty spots between the cantaloupe points.

6. Then place ¼ of the cabbage mixture in the empty space in the middle of the X. Top with ¼ of the chopped walnuts. Serve immediately.

PER SERVING | Calories: 166 | Fat: 5 g | Protein: 3 g | Sodium: 36 mg | Fiber: 4 g | Carbohydrates: 30 g | Sugar: 24 g

Thai Pasta Salad

*Colorful fresh veggies and the flavors of sesame and ginger make this
hearty pasta salad a treat. Serve warm or cold.*

INGREDIENTS | SERVES 8

1 (16-ounce) package dry spaghetti

2 tablespoons peanut oil

1 medium yellow squash, julienned

1 medium zucchini, julienned

1 medium green bell pepper, julienned

1 red bell pepper, julienned

1 orange bell pepper, julienned

6 scallions, sliced

3 cloves garlic, minced

1 jalapeño pepper, minced

¾ cup chopped walnuts

⅓ cup peanut oil

1 tablespoon sesame oil

¼ cup unflavored rice vinegar

2 tablespoons salt-free peanut butter

1 tablespoon no-salt-added tomato paste

¼ cup chopped fresh cilantro

1 tablespoon minced fresh ginger

1 teaspoon sugar

¼ teaspoon salt-free chili seasoning

1. Bring a large pot of water to boil over high heat. Once boiling, break the spaghetti in half and add to the pot. Cook for 10 minutes, stirring once or twice. Remove from heat, drain, and set aside.

2. Heat 2 tablespoons peanut oil in a large sauté pan over medium heat. Add the julienned vegetables, scallions, garlic, jalapeño, and walnuts and cook, stirring, for 3–4 minutes.

3. Remove from heat and transfer to a very large bowl. Add cooked spaghetti.

4. Whisk the remaining ingredients together in a mixing bowl. Pour over the pasta salad and toss well to coat. Serve immediately or cover and refrigerate until ready to serve.

PER SERVING | Calories: 464 | Fat: 24 g | Protein: 11 g | Sodium: 9 mg | Fiber: 5 g | Carbohydrates: 50 g | Sugar: 4 g

Whole-Wheat Couscous Salad with Citrus and Cilantro

This whole-grain salad strikes the perfect balance between light and filling. Its refreshing taste can be enjoyed year round, but is best in summer with produce picked fresh from the garden.

INGREDIENTS | SERVES 6

1½ cups water

1 cup whole-wheat couscous

1 medium cucumber

1 pint grape or cherry tomatoes, halved

1 jalapeño pepper, minced

2 shallots, minced

2 scallions, sliced

2 cloves garlic, minced

2 tablespoons freshly squeezed lemon juice

2 tablespoons freshly squeezed lime juice

1 teaspoon olive oil

¼ cup chopped fresh cilantro

Freshly ground black pepper, to taste

1. Measure water into a saucepan and bring to a boil over high heat. Once boiling, stir in the couscous, reduce heat to medium-low, cover, and simmer for 2 minutes.

2. Remove pot from heat, remove lid, and fluff couscous with a fork. Set aside to cool for 5 minutes.

3. Peel the cucumber and slice in half lengthwise. Use a spoon to gently scrape out the seeds, then dice and place into a mixing bowl.

4. Add the remaining ingredients to the bowl along with the cooked couscous and toss well to coat.

5. Season to taste with freshly ground black pepper. Serve immediately or cover and refrigerate until ready to serve.

PER SERVING | Calories: 126 | Fat: 2 g | Protein: 4 g | Sodium: 5 mg | Fiber: 2 g | Carbohydrates: 24 g | Sugar: 3 g

What Is Couscous?

Couscous is a tiny grain-like pasta made from semolina (wheat) flour. It cooks in minutes and makes an easy and convenient alternative to rice and other grains. Couscous comes in white and whole-wheat varieties; the whole-wheat version has the added benefits of whole grain, thus making it a healthier choice. Couscous is low in fat and sodium and is a good source of protein, fiber, and iron. It's sold in most supermarkets and natural food stores, both in packages and dry bulk bins, and is often stocked alongside rice and other grains.

Salad Niçoise

The famous French salad, low-sodium style. Delightful and impressive, it's a plate full of color, flavor, and protein with a dreamy dressing that pulls it all together. The salad has several cooking steps; boil ingredients simultaneously to speed preparation.

INGREDIENTS | SERVES 2

1 small head butter lettuce
1 small cucumber
2 medium red potatoes
1 tablespoon white distilled vinegar
2 eggs
1 bunch fresh green beans, trimmed
2 tablespoons olive oil
2 tablespoons red wine vinegar
1 teaspoon salt-free prepared mustard
1 clove garlic, minced
½ teaspoon freshly ground black pepper
2 small tomatoes, quartered
1 (5-ounce) can no-salt-added tuna in water, drained

1. Wash the lettuce and pat dry. Tear the leaves into bite-sized pieces and set aside.

2. Peel the cucumber, halve lengthwise, and remove seeds using a spoon. Slice and set aside.

3. Place the potatoes into a pan and add enough water to cover. Bring to a boil over high heat, then reduce heat slightly, and simmer until tender, about 20 minutes. Once cooked, dice, toss with white vinegar, and set aside.

4. Place the eggs into a saucepan, add enough water to cover, and bring to a boil over high heat. Boil 12 minutes. Once cooked, carefully crack, peel, and slice into quarters. Set aside.

5. Bring a small pot of water to boil. Once boiling, add the green beans and cook for 2 minutes. Remove beans from pot and immediately place in a bowl of ice water. Set aside.

6. In a small bowl, add the oil, vinegar, mustard, garlic, and pepper and whisk well to combine.

7. Assemble the salad on a platter, placing lettuce on the bottom and then grouping the cucumber, potatoes, eggs, green beans, tomatoes, and tuna on top. Drizzle the dressing evenly over the salad. Serve immediately.

PER SERVING | Calories: 471 | Fat: 20 g | Protein: 30 g | Sodium: 111 mg | Fiber: 7 g | Carbohydrates: 41 g | Sugar: 5 g

Simple Autumn Salad

*A tasty combination of red leaf lettuce, red onion, fruit, and walnuts in a
light and tangy vinaigrette. Salt free, healthy, and delicious.*

INGREDIENTS | SERVES 4

1 large head red leaf lettuce

1 pear, thinly sliced

½ small red onion, thinly sliced

½ cup dried black mission figs, chopped

⅓ cup chopped walnuts

2 tablespoons white balsamic vinegar

2 tablespoons olive oil

1 clove garlic, minced

¼ teaspoon freshly ground black pepper

1. Wash the lettuce, pat dry, then tear into bite-sized pieces. Place in a bowl with the sliced pear, onion, figs, and walnuts. Set aside.

2. In a small bowl, add the vinegar, oil, garlic, and black pepper and whisk well to combine. Pour the dressing over the salad and toss to coat. Serve immediately.

PER SERVING | Calories: 224 | Fat: 14 g | Protein: 3 g | Sodium: 29 mg | Fiber: 5 g | Carbohydrates: 25 g | Sugar: 15 g

Stock Up and Save

There's nothing more irritating than running out of a crucial ingredient when you're ready to cook. And this goes doubly when you're on a specialized diet and don't have the luxury of ordering out. By buying items in bulk, you'll not only be saving money, as per unit costs are often cheaper, you'll also be hedging against future inconvenience.

Rice Salad with Black Beans, Mango, and Lime

*Delicious warm or cold, this salad showcases simple, fresh flavors the best way possible: naked!
Use whichever rice you prefer—brown, basmati, jasmine, even wild rice—all work well.*

INGREDIENTS | SERVES 6

3 cups cooked rice

1 (15-ounce) can no-salt-added black beans, drained

1 ripe mango, diced

1 medium red bell pepper, diced

2 scallions, sliced

2 cloves garlic, minced

Juice of 2 fresh limes

¼ cup chopped fresh cilantro

Freshly ground black pepper, to taste

1. Place all the ingredients into a mixing bowl and stir well to combine.

2. Serve immediately or cover and refrigerate until ready to serve.

PER SERVING | Calories: 230 | Fat: 1 g | Protein: 9 g | Sodium: 4 mg | Fiber: 7 g | Carbohydrates: 47 g | Sugar: 6 g

Apple Carrot Salad with Cider Vinaigrette

*This delightful salad makes a great light meal or filling for wrap sandwiches.
The sweetness of the carrot and apple contrasts the tartness of the vinegar and
the lively zing of the garlic, scallion, and parsley. The flavor improves as the ingredients
marinate, so make this ahead of time, even the day before. Adapted from Vegetarian Times.*

INGREDIENTS | SERVES 4

2 tablespoons apple cider vinegar

1 tablespoon olive oil

1 clove garlic, minced

1 teaspoon agave nectar

2 medium carrots, grated

1 small apple, diced

2 scallions, sliced

¼ cup chopped fresh parsley

¼ cup dried cranberries

Freshly ground black pepper, to taste

4 cups fresh baby spinach

1. Add the vinegar, oil, garlic, and agave nectar to a small bowl and whisk well to combine.

2. Place the carrots, apple, scallions, parsley, and cranberries into a mixing bowl.

3. Pour the dressing over top and toss well to coat. Season to taste with freshly ground black pepper. Cover and refrigerate until ready to serve.

4. When ready to serve, arrange baby spinach on 4 plates and divide salad evenly over top. Serve immediately.

PER SERVING | Calories: 112 | Fat: 3 g | Protein: 1 g | Sodium: 46 mg | Fiber: 3 g | Carbohydrates: 20 g | Sugar: 14 g

Tuna Pasta Salad with Broccoli and Sundried Tomatoes

Bold flavors combine flawlessly in this healthy salt-free salad. With whole grain, low-fat protein, vitamins, and nutrients, it's a one-dish meal that's wonderful served warm or cold.

INGREDIENTS | SERVES 8

½ cup chopped sundried tomatoes (not in oil)

1 cup boiling water

1 (13-ounce) package dry whole-grain penne

1 tablespoon olive oil

1 head broccoli, cut into small florets

2 shallots, finely diced

2 (5-ounce) cans no-salt-added tuna in water, drained

2 tablespoons balsamic vinegar

½ teaspoon freshly ground black pepper

What Is Vinegar?

Vinegar is produced when an alcoholic liquid is allowed to ferment and the ethanol within it oxidizes. The remaining liquid becomes highly acidic, and is what we refer to as vinegar. Balsamic vinegar is made from the leftover pressings, or must, of white grapes that are first boiled down to form a syrup then allowed to age. Apple cider vinegar is made from a similar process using apple must.

1. Place sundried tomatoes in a bowl, add water, and let soak for 10 minutes. Reserve 2 tablespoons of liquid.

2. Cook penne according to package directions, omitting salt. Drain and set aside.

3. Heat 1 tablespoon oil in a sauté pan. Add the broccoli and sauté for 5 minutes.

4. Remove from heat. Add the sundried tomatoes, 2 tablespoons of the tomato soaking liquid, penne, shallots, tuna, vinegar, and black pepper to the pan and stir well to combine.

5. Serve immediately or cover and refrigerate until ready to serve.

PER SERVING | Calories: 233 | Fat: 3 g | Protein: 16 g | Sodium: 107 mg | Fiber: 7 g | Carbohydrates: 36 g | Sugar: 3 g

Sweet Potato Salad with Maple Vinaigrette

In one word: YUM! This hearty salad makes a healthy and filling one-dish meal. For more color, add a small handful of dried cherries or cranberries.

INGREDIENTS | SERVES 6

4 small–medium sweet potatoes

1 (15-ounce) can no-salt-added garbanzo beans

4 scallions, sliced

1 shallot, minced

2 tablespoons pure maple syrup

2 tablespoons freshly squeezed lemon juice

1½ teaspoons olive oil

½ teaspoon dry ground mustard

¼ teaspoon freshly ground black pepper

Southwestern Sweet Potato Salad

For a spicier version of this salad, try the following. Instead of using garbanzos, substitute an equal amount of black beans. Add minced garlic instead of shallot, omit the mustard, and swap lime juice for the lemon. Add a teaspoon of ground cumin and another of salt-free chili seasoning. Stir in a handful of chopped fresh cilantro and serve!

1. Place unpeeled sweet potatoes into a pot and add enough water to cover by a couple of inches. Bring to a boil over high heat and simmer until tender, about 20 minutes.

2. Remove pot from heat and drain. Place the sweet potatoes under cold running water until cool enough to handle, then peel, and cut into chunks.

3. Place sweet potatoes into a mixing bowl, along with the beans, scallions, and shallot.

4. Whisk together the remaining ingredients in a small bowl and pour over salad. Toss gently to coat.

5. Serve immediately or cover and refrigerate until ready to serve.

PER SERVING | Calories: 224 | Fat: 3 g | Protein: 7 g | Sodium: 33 mg | Fiber: 8 g | Carbohydrates: 42 g | Sugar: 13 g

Arugula with Pears and Red Wine Vinaigrette

The peppery taste of arugula is partnered with crisp, sweet pears and a tangy red wine vinaigrette. Add grilled chicken, chopped nuts, dried figs, and/or shredded cheese for a main-course salad.

INGREDIENTS | SERVES 4

8 cups fresh baby arugula
2 pears, sliced thinly
4 tablespoons red wine vinegar
2 tablespoons olive oil
1 clove garlic, minced
½ teaspoon dried marjoram
¼ teaspoon dry ground mustard
¼ teaspoon freshly ground black pepper

1. Place the arugula into a large mixing bowl and add the sliced pears.

2. Add the remaining ingredients to a small mixing bowl and whisk well to combine.

3. Pour over salad and toss well to coat. Serve immediately.

PER SERVING | Calories: 127 | Fat: 7 g | Protein: 1 g | Sodium: 13 mg | Fiber: 3 g | Carbohydrates: 15 g | Sugar: 9 g

Tomato Cucumber Basil Salad

Ripe, garden-fresh produce in a tangy vinaigrette. It's like savoring a bowl full of summer.

INGREDIENTS | SERVES 4

2 small–medium cucumbers
4 ripe medium tomatoes, quartered
1 small onion, sliced thinly
¼ cup chopped fresh basil
3 tablespoons red wine vinegar
1 tablespoon olive oil
1 clove garlic, minced
¼ teaspoon freshly ground black pepper

1. Peel the cucumbers. Halve lengthwise, then use a spoon to gently scrape out the seeds.

2. Slice cucumbers and place in a bowl. Add the tomatoes, onion, and basil.

3. Place the remaining ingredients into a small bowl and whisk well to combine.

4. Pour the dressing over the salad and toss to coat. Serve immediately or cover and refrigerate until ready to serve.

PER SERVING | Calories: 66 | Fat: 4 g | Protein: 1 g | Sodium: 9 mg | Fiber: 2 g | Carbohydrates: 7 g | Sugar: 4 g

Curried Tofu Salad

A curried twist on Waldorf salad, this vegan version adds the heft and protein of tofu and swaps mayonnaise for a lighter vinaigrette. Adapted from Eating Well When You Just Can't Eat The Way You Used To.

INGREDIENTS | SERVES 6

1 pound extra-firm tofu, drained and cubed

3 medium stalks celery, diced

1 small green apple, diced

1 small red apple, cored and diced

¾ cup golden raisins

¼ cup chopped walnuts

3 tablespoons apple cider vinegar

2 tablespoons canola oil

1 teaspoon salt-free curry powder

⅛ teaspoon ground cumin

⅛ teaspoon ground white pepper

Tofu Safety

When buying tofu sold in water, whether it's sold in a sealed container or not, it's important to steam it for several minutes before eating it raw. The steaming process will kill any active bacteria and save you from potential sickness. Tofu that is sold in sealed, shelf-stable packaging does not need to be steamed before it's eaten raw; this type of tofu has already gone through a pasteurization process.

1. Place the tofu into the steamer basket of a pot or appliance and steam for 5 minutes. Remove and set aside to cool.

2. Place the celery, apples, raisins, and walnuts into a mixing bowl and add tofu when it has cooled to touch.

3. Measure the remaining ingredients into a small bowl and whisk well to combine. Drizzle the dressing over the salad and toss gently to coat.

4. Serve immediately or cover and refrigerate until ready to serve.

PER SERVING | Calories: 226 | Fat: 12 g | Protein: 9 g | Sodium: 22 mg | Fiber: 3 g | Carbohydrates: 23 g | Sugar: 15 g

Strawberry Vinaigrette

Sweet with a smidgen of tart acidity, so much flavor, and zero salt. This dressing is a beautiful complement to every salad, from greens to fruit. But don't stop there. Try this with grilled meat, even drizzled over cake! Adapted from Simply in Season.

INGREDIENTS | YIELDS 1½ CUPS

1 cup sliced fresh strawberries

4 teaspoons unflavored rice vinegar

4 teaspoons freshly squeezed lemon juice

1 tablespoon sugar

1½ teaspoons honey

⅛ teaspoon garlic powder

⅛ teaspoon onion powder

⅛ teaspoon dried basil

⅛ teaspoon freshly ground black pepper

4 tablespoons olive oil

1. Place the sliced strawberries into a blender or food processor and pulse until smooth.

2. Add all the remaining ingredients except the oil and blend.

3. Gradually add the oil and pulse until combined.

4. Use immediately or store in an airtight container and refrigerate. Use within 2 days.

PER SERVING (2 TABLESPOONS) | Calories: 53 | Fat: 4 g | Protein: 0 g | Sodium: 0 mg | Fiber: 0 g | Carbohydrates: 3 g | Sugar: 2 g

What Is Honey?

Honey is a liquid sweetener made when honey bees consume nectar and bring it back to their hive. As the bees transport the nectar from flower to hive, it mixes with special enzymes in their saliva, forming honey. Although this may sound less than appealing, honey is anything but. Apart from its amazing taste, raw honey is said to help heal wounds and infections, protect against allergies, and even inhibit disease.

Pomegranate Balsamic Vinaigrette

The deep flavors of pomegranate and balsamic vinegar are natural complements.
Serve this dressing over simple greens with sliced fruit, grilled meat, and a little grated cheese.

INGREDIENTS | YIELDS ½ CUP

3 tablespoons pomegranate juice (e.g., Pom)
3 tablespoons balsamic vinegar
1 tablespoon olive oil
2 cloves garlic, minced
½ teaspoon dried herbes de Provence
Freshly ground black pepper, to taste

1. Place all the ingredients into a small mixing bowl and whisk well to combine.

2. Use immediately or cover and refrigerate until ready to serve. If stored, whisk again before serving.

PER SERVING (2 TABLESPOONS) | Calories: 50 | Fat: 3 g | Protein: 0 g | Sodium: 4 mg | Fiber: 0 g | Carbohydrates: 4 g | Sugar: 3 g

Lemon Vinaigrette

Get ready to lick your plate! This irresistibly zesty dressing adds sparkle to salads
and makes a great marinade for veggies, meat, and tofu.

INGREDIENTS | YIELDS 3 OUNCES

¼ cup freshly squeezed lemon juice
1 tablespoon olive oil
1 tablespoon minced fresh shallot
1 tablespoon honey
⅛ teaspoon ground white pepper

1. Place all the ingredients into a small bowl and whisk well to combine.

2. Use immediately or cover and refrigerate until ready to serve.

PER SERVING (1 OUNCE) | Calories: 69 | Fat: 4 g | Protein: 0 g | Sodium: 0 mg | Fiber: 0 g | Carbohydrates: 8 g | Sugar: 6 g

Quick Twists

Substitute lime or key lime, grapefruit, orange, or tangerine juice for the lemon juice in this vinaigrette. Add a tablespoon of chopped fresh mint. Trade minced ginger or sliced scallion for the shallot. Use agave nectar instead of the honey.

Apple Honey Mustard Vinaigrette

Toss this tart, tangy, absolutely delicious dressing with salad greens or use as a base for sautéed spinach, Swiss chard, or kale.

INGREDIENTS | YIELDS ½ CUP

¼ cup apple cider vinegar
2 tablespoons honey
1 tablespoon olive oil
1 teaspoon dry ground mustard
⅛ teaspoon ground white pepper

1. Place all the ingredients into a small bowl and whisk well to combine.

2. Serve immediately or cover and refrigerate until ready to serve.

PER SERVING (2 TABLESPOONS) | Calories: 65 | Fat: 3 g | Protein: 0 g | Sodium: 1 mg | Fiber: 0 g | Carbohydrates: 9 g | Sugar: 8 g

Italian Vinaigrette

A simple all-purpose salad dressing that also works well as a marinade.

INGREDIENTS | YIELDS ¼ CUP

3 tablespoons white distilled vinegar
1½ teaspoons olive oil
2 cloves garlic, minced
½ teaspoon dried Italian seasoning
½ teaspoon all-purpose salt-free seasoning

1. Place all the ingredients into a small bowl and whisk well to combine.

2. Serve immediately or cover and refrigerate until ready to serve.

PER SERVING (2 TABLESPOONS) | Calories: 37 | Fat: 3 g | Protein: 0 g | Sodium: 1 mg | Fiber: 0 g | Carbohydrates: 1 g | Sugar: 0 g

Own Your Own Health

Transitioning to a healthy diet often requires dramatic changes in thought and behavior. A good way to encourage yourself is to leave reminders around the house. Tape small notes to the outside and inside of the refrigerator, for example, reminding you of the importance of healthy choices. It's easy to lose sight of these things, especially when you're hungry.

Sesame Ginger Vinaigrette

*Modeled after the dressings served at many Japanese restaurants,
this low-sodium vinaigrette will have you craving salads like never before.*

INGREDIENTS | YIELDS ⅓ CUP

¼ cup unflavored rice wine vinegar
1 tablespoon sesame oil
1 tablespoon minced fresh ginger
2 cloves garlic, minced
1 teaspoon sugar
¼ teaspoon ground white pepper

1. Place all of the ingredients into a small microwave-safe bowl and whisk well to combine.

2. Place in the microwave for 30 seconds, remove, and whisk well again.

3. Pour over salad and toss well to coat. Serve immediately.

PER SERVING (2 TABLESPOONS) | Calories: 58 | Fat: 5 g | Protein: 0 g | Sodium: 0 mg | Fiber: 0 g | Carbohydrates: 2 g | Sugar: 1 g

Tomato Garlic Dressing

If you're someone who puts ketchup on everything, here's the dressing of your dreams! With its vibrant color and tangy taste, it's great drizzled over salad or served with grilled vegetables, meats, and sandwiches.

INGREDIENTS | YIELDS ⅓ CUP

2 tablespoons red wine vinegar

2 tablespoons lemon juice

1 tablespoon salt-free tomato paste

1½ teaspoons olive oil

2 cloves garlic

1 teaspoon agave nectar

⅛ teaspoon ground white pepper

1. Place all of the ingredients into a food processor and pulse until smooth.

2. Serve immediately or store in an airtight container until ready to serve.

PER SERVING (2 TABLESPOONS) | Calories: 60 | Fat: 2 g | Protein: 0 g | Sodium: 7 mg | Fiber: 0 g | Carbohydrates: 9 g | Sugar: 7 g

Homemade Dressing

Store-bought salad dressings offer convenience, but at what cost? Most are filled with fat, excess sodium, and unrecognizable ingredients. Instead of buying commercial dressings, spend money on new and interesting vinegars, oils, and fruit juices. Add garlic, scallions, or shallot, fresh or dried herbs, ground or prepared mustard, some spice, and you've got a world of flavor in minutes.

Vegan Caesar Salad Dressing

With undertones of garlic and lemon, this smooth and creamy dressing provides all of the flavor of the classic without the cholesterol. Toss with crisp romaine lettuce and Salt-Free Croutons (see Chapter 3) or serve as a dip with raw veggies.

INGREDIENTS | YIELDS ¼ CUP

¼ cup pine nuts or walnuts

¼ cup low-sodium vegetable broth

2 cloves garlic

1 tablespoon freshly squeezed lemon juice

¼ teaspoon dry ground mustard

⅛ teaspoon ground white pepper

1. Place all of the ingredients into a food processor and pulse until smooth.

2. Serve immediately.

PER SERVING (2 TABLESPOONS) | Calories: 106 | Fat: 10 g | Protein: 3 g | Sodium: 10 mg | Fiber: 1 g | Carbohydrates: 4 g | Sugar: 0 g

Soups, Stews, and Chilis

Apple Butternut Soup

Apples draw out the natural sweetness of butternut squash,
delivering a smooth, irresistibly delicious fat-free soup.

INGREDIENTS | SERVES 6

6 cups diced butternut squash

2 cups diced apple

6 cups water

2 cups unsweetened apple juice ·

½ teaspoon ground cinnamon

⅛ teaspoon ground allspice

Apple Facts

Apples are one of the most widely consumed fruits in the world. They can be eaten raw, cooked, dried, juiced, or fermented, without diminishing their nutritional value. For best health, buy organic apples, wash, and consume along with the skin. The peel provides added nutrients and fiber. Apples contain vitamins C and K as well as flavanoids, substances believed to prevent cancer.

1. Placed diced squash and apple into a stockpot, add the water and juice, and bring to a boil over high heat. Once boiling, reduce heat to medium-low, cover, and simmer for 20 minutes.

2. Remove from heat and purée using a blender or food processor.

3. Return soup to the pot, add spices, and stir to combine. Serve warm.

PER SERVING | Calories: 150 | Fat: 0 g | Protein: 3 g | Sodium: 8 mg | Fiber: 1 g | Carbohydrates: 38 g | Sugar: 11 g

Banana Coconut Soup with Tropical Fruit

*This sublime soup offers a taste of paradise in mere minutes.
Serve as a cool starter, light dessert, or lovely addition to breakfast.*

INGREDIENTS | SERVES 4

2 medium ripe bananas

1 (14-ounce) can light coconut milk

1 tablespoon honey

⅛ teaspoon ground cardamom

1 ripe mango, diced

1 ripe kiwi, sliced

2 cups cubed fresh pineapple

1. Peel the bananas, place in a food processor, and purée.

2. Add the coconut milk and pulse to combine.

3. Pour contents of food processor into a small mixing bowl. Add the honey and cardamom and stir to combine.

4. Divide evenly between 4 bowls, then top with fresh fruit. Serve immediately.

PER SERVING | Calories: 235 | Fat: 7 g | Protein: 1 g | Sodium: 24 mg | Fiber: 4 g | Carbohydrates: 42 g | Sugar: 31 g

Easy Wonton Soup

*This low-sodium soup mimics classic wonton so much, you'll be hard pressed to tell the difference.
Add your choice of fresh mushrooms, from basic white button or baby bella to oyster or shitake.*

INGREDIENTS | SERVES 8

½ pound lean ground pork

1 tablespoon minced fresh ginger

4 cloves garlic, minced

8 cups low-sodium chicken broth

2 cups sliced fresh mushrooms

6 ounces dry whole-grain yolk-free egg noodles

¼ teaspoon ground white pepper

4 scallions, sliced

1. Place a stockpot over medium heat. Add the ground pork, ginger, and garlic and sauté for 5 minutes. Drain any excess fat, then return to stovetop over medium heat.

2. Add the broth and bring to a boil. Once boiling, stir in the mushrooms, noodles, and white pepper. Cover and simmer for 10 minutes.

3. Remove pot from heat. Stir in the scallions and serve immediately.

PER SERVING | Calories: 143 | Fat: 4 g | Protein: 12 g | Sodium: 90 mg | Fiber: 1 g | Carbohydrates: 14 g | Sugar: 1 g

Carrot Soup with Ginger

Bursting with vitamin A, this fat-free soup gets an A+ for its delightful taste and fabulous color.

INGREDIENTS | SERVES 4

4 cups diced carrot

1 cup diced sweet potato

1 cup diced sweet onion

4 cups low-sodium vegetable or chicken broth

1 tablespoon minced fresh ginger

2 tablespoons chopped fresh parsley

Carrot Facts

Vibrant, crunchy, and sweetly delicious, carrots are a beloved vegetable among humans and animals alike. They can be eaten raw, cooked, or juiced. Carrots contain high levels of vitamin A and antioxidants, and are believed to help prevent cancer.

1. Combine carrot, sweet potato, onion, broth, and ginger in a small stockpot and bring to a boil over high heat. Once boiling, reduce heat to low and simmer, covered, for 30 minutes.

2. Remove from heat and purée using a blender or food processor. Serve immediately, garnished with parsley.

PER SERVING | Calories: 163 | Fat: 2 g | Protein: 7 g | Sodium: 86 mg | Fiber: 6 g | Carbohydrates: 32 g | Sugar: 13 g

Black Bean Vegetable Soup

Thick and hearty, with a deep rich taste, this fat-free vegetarian soup is ready in under 30 minutes. Don't drain the canned tomatoes or beans; the liquid becomes part of the flavorful stock.

INGREDIENTS | SERVES 4

2½ cups low-sodium vegetable broth

1 small red onion, diced

3 cloves garlic, minced

1 small carrot, diced

1 small stalk celery, diced

1 small sweet potato, diced

1 (15-ounce) can no-salt-added diced tomatoes

1 (15-ounce) can no-salt-added black beans

¼ cup red wine

1 tablespoon no-salt-added tomato paste

1½ teaspoons ground cumin

1 teaspoon dried oregano

½ teaspoon ground coriander

¼ teaspoon dried red pepper flakes

Freshly ground black pepper, to taste

2 tablespoons chopped fresh cilantro

1. Place a stockpot over medium heat. Add ¼ cup of the vegetable broth, onion, and garlic and sauté for 2 minutes.

2. Add another ¼ cup broth, carrot, celery, sweet potato, and tomatoes with juice and sauté for 3 minutes.

3. Add remaining ingredients, except cilantro. Bring to a boil, cover, and simmer for 15–20 minutes, until veggies are tender.

4. Remove from heat, stir in the cilantro, and serve immediately.

PER SERVING | Calories: 233 | Fat: 2 g | Protein: 10 g | Sodium: 88 mg | Fiber: 8 g | Carbohydrates: 41 g | Sugar: 6 g

Basic Low-Sodium Broth

A fat-free vegan broth perfect for flavoring your favorite soup or sipping straight from a mug.

INGREDIENTS | YIELDS 8 CUPS

1 medium yellow onion, peeled
3 garlic cloves, peeled
8 ounces mushrooms, scrubbed
3 medium carrots, scrubbed
2 medium stalks celery, scrubbed
2 medium tomatoes
1-inch piece fresh ginger
6 whole peppercorns
2 bay leaves
10 cups water

Homemade Versus Commercial Broth

Homemade broth is often tastier than store bought, and it's also additive and preservative free. Homemade broth can be made in batches and frozen for later use. When pressed for time, however, commercial low-sodium broths can be a good alternative, as long as they're also low in fat. Check nutrition facts carefully; some manufacturers sell "reduced sodium" broths that contain hundreds of mg per serving. Some excellent commercial broths are made by Pacific Foods, Imagine Foods, and Kitchen Basics.

1. Quarter the onion, garlic cloves, and mushrooms. Slice the carrots, celery, and tomatoes into chunks. Place into a stockpot, along with all the remaining ingredients.

2. Cover pot and bring to a boil over high heat. Once boiling, reduce heat to medium-low and simmer for 30 minutes.

3. Turn off the heat and let the contents steep for another 30 minutes.

4. Pour broth through a fine mesh sieve, discarding the vegetables. Use immediately, store in the refrigerator for up to a week, or freeze.

PER SERVING | Calories: 12 | Fat: 0 g | Protein: 0 g | Sodium: 9 mg | Fiber: 0 g | Carbohydrates: 3 g | Sugar: 2 g

Cheesy Potato Chowder

This creamy, dreamy concoction of potatoes, chicken broth, and cheese will make a low-sodium soup fan of even the staunchest critic.

INGREDIENTS | SERVES 6

1 tablespoon olive oil
2 cups diced onion
1 cup diced celery
2 cloves garlic, minced
6 cups diced potato
4 cups low-sodium chicken broth
⅓ cup dry white wine
½ teaspoon dried thyme
¼ teaspoon ground rosemary
⅛ teaspoon dried basil
Freshly ground black pepper, to taste
1 cup shredded Swiss cheese

1. Heat oil in a stockpot over medium. Add onion, celery, and garlic and sauté for 5 minutes.

2. Add potato and cook, stirring, for 1 minute. Add the broth, white wine, herbs, and black pepper, to taste.

3. Bring to a boil. Once boiling, reduce heat to low, cover, and simmer for 20 minutes.

4. Remove pot from heat. Using a blender or food processor, purée roughly half the soup. Return soup to pot and stir well to combine.

5. Add the shredded cheese and stir until melted.

6. Ladle the chowder into bowls and garnish with additional Swiss cheese, if desired. Serve hot.

PER SERVING | Calories: 252 | Fat: 8 g | Protein: 11 g | Sodium: 94 mg | Fiber: 3 g | Carbohydrates: 33 g | Sugar: 3 g

Chicken Soup with Jalapeño and Lime

Set your taste buds abuzz with the zing of fresh lime! This low-sodium soup is brimming over with flavor, yet virtually fat free. For added heft, ladle soup over bowls of cooked brown or wild rice.

INGREDIENTS | SERVES 8

2 cups cooked, shredded chicken

1 medium red onion, diced

3 cloves garlic, minced

2 medium carrots, sliced

1 medium stalk celery, sliced

1 medium red bell pepper, diced

1 jalapeño pepper, minced

1 (15-ounce) can no-salt-added diced tomatoes

Juice of 2 fresh limes

8 cups low-sodium chicken broth

1 teaspoon ground cumin

½ teaspoon ground coriander

¼ teaspoon dried oregano

Freshly ground black pepper, to taste

2 tablespoons chopped fresh cilantro

1 fresh lime, cut into wedges

1. Place all the ingredients except cilantro and lime wedges into a stockpot and bring to a boil over high heat.

2. Once boiling, reduce heat to low, cover, and simmer for 15 minutes.

3. Remove from heat, ladle into bowls, and garnish with chopped cilantro and lime wedges. Serve immediately.

PER SERVING | Calories: 118 | Fat: 2 g | Protein: 6 g | Sodium: 111 mg | Fiber: 1 g | Carbohydrates: 9 g | Sugar: 3 g

Hot, Hot, Hot!

Hot peppers, or chili peppers, add tremendous dimension to food without upping the sodium ante. Hot peppers come in many colorful varieties and vary widely in heat, from the fairly mild jalapeño to the nearly intolerable Scotch bonnet. Hot peppers are easy to grow in the garden, and can be preserved through freezing or drying. To freeze, simply seal in an airtight container and freeze for up to a year. To dry peppers, place on a flat surface until they shrivel and dehydrate, or string them and hang to dry.

Classic Chicken Noodle Soup

No cookbook would be complete without this perennial favorite.
This low-fat, low-sodium version makes the most of meaty chicken and tender veggies.

INGREDIENTS | SERVES 4

2 cups cooked, shredded chicken

2 medium carrots, sliced

1 medium stalk celery, sliced

1 small onion, diced

3 cloves garlic, minced

4 cups low-sodium chicken broth

1 teaspoon all-purpose salt-free seasoning

½ teaspoon ground sage

¼ teaspoon ground rosemary

Freshly ground black pepper, to taste

1½ cups yolkless egg noodles

1. Combine all the ingredients except noodles in a stockpot. Bring to a boil over high heat.

2. Once boiling, add the noodles, reduce heat to medium-low, and simmer 10 minutes.

3. Remove from heat. Ladle soup into bowls and serve immediately.

PER SERVING | Calories: 291 | Fat: 5 g | Protein: 33 g | Sodium: 167 mg | Fiber: 2 g | Carbohydrates: 26 g | Sugar: 2 g

Garden Tomato Soup

Ripe tomatoes, sweet bell pepper, and onion partner perfectly in this fresh vegetable soup. Serve with grilled Swiss cheese sandwiches for a sensational low-sodium meal.

INGREDIENTS | SERVES 4

1 tablespoon olive oil

3 cups chopped, peeled, and seeded tomatoes

1 cup chopped onion

1 cup chopped red bell pepper

1 tablespoon minced garlic

4 cups low-sodium vegetable broth

2 tablespoons no-salt-added tomato paste

1 tablespoon chopped fresh basil

1 teaspoon chopped fresh oregano

½ teaspoon chopped fresh thyme

Freshly ground black pepper, to taste

1. Heat the oil in a stockpot over medium heat. Add the tomatoes, onion, bell pepper, and garlic and cook, stirring, for 10 minutes.

2. Add the remaining ingredients and stir to combine. Raise heat to high and bring to a boil.

3. Once boiling, reduce heat to low, cover, and simmer for 10 minutes.

4. Remove from heat and purée using a blender or food processor. Serve immediately.

PER SERVING | Calories: 130 | Fat: 5 g | Protein: 3 g | Sodium: 20 mg | Fiber: 2 g | Carbohydrates: 19 g | Sugar: 4 g

Tips to Reduce Dietary Sodium

Use fresh, local, organic produce whenever possible. Fresh fruits and vegetables have not been processed, meaning nothing has been added to them, including salt. By buying organic produce, you protect yourself from the risks associated with harmful chemical pesticides and fertilizers. And by supporting local farmers, you ensure their livelihood and the continuation of the food stock you enjoy.

Hearty Vegetable Beef Soup

A great remedy for chilly winter weather, this no-nonsense recipe comes together in 30 minutes with ingredients many people already have on hand.

INGREDIENTS | SERVES 8

1 pound lean ground beef

1 large onion, diced

3 medium carrots, sliced

3 medium stalks celery, sliced

6 cloves garlic, minced

1 (15-ounce) can no-salt-added diced tomatoes

1 (8-ounce) can no-salt-added tomato sauce

4 cups low-sodium beef broth

2 teaspoons dried Italian seasoning

Freshly ground black pepper, to taste

1. Brown ground beef in a stockpot over medium heat. Once beef is cooked, carefully drain out any excess fat.

2. Add remaining ingredients to the pot, raise heat to high, and bring to a boil.

3. Once boiling, reduce heat to low, cover, and simmer for 25–30 minutes, stirring occasionally.

4. Remove from heat and serve immediately.

PER SERVING | Calories: 121 | Fat: 3 g | Protein: 13 g | Sodium: 85 mg | Fiber: 2 g | Carbohydrates: 11 g | Sugar: 5 g

Kale Soup with Lemon and Tuna

The citrus kiss of this healthy soup brings sunshine to the darkest days. No-salt-added canned tuna adds protein and omega-3 fatty acids. Substitute another cooked fish if desired or omit for a strictly vegetarian soup.

INGREDIENTS | SERVES 4

1 teaspoon olive oil

1 large shallot, minced

3 cloves garlic, minced

Juice of 2 fresh lemons

8 cups chopped fresh kale

4 cups low-sodium chicken or vegetable broth

2 (5-ounce) cans no-salt-added tuna, in water

¼ cup wheat berries, uncooked

1 teaspoon salt-free herbes de Provence

Freshly ground black pepper, to taste

1. Heat oil in a stockpot over medium heat. Add the shallot and garlic and sauté for 2 minutes.

2. Add lemon juice and kale and cook, stirring, until kale has wilted, about 2 minutes.

3. Add the remaining ingredients and cover. Raise heat to high and bring to a boil. Once boiling, reduce heat to low and simmer for 20 minutes.

4. Remove from heat and serve immediately.

PER SERVING | Calories: 264 | Fat: 5 g | Protein: 28 g | Sodium: 166 mg | Fiber: 5 g | Carbohydrates: 29 g | Sugar: 1 g

Canned Tuna Concern

Studies show that many brand name tunas often exceed the FDA's advisory limits for mercury and should not be consumed with regularity. If you are buying supermarket tuna, opt for chunk light over white albacore, as the light tuna is lower in mercury. Some premium tuna brands, such as Oregon's Choice, contain far lower levels of mercury and higher values of omega-3s. Oregon's Choice Gourmet No Salt Added Albacore Tuna can be purchased online.

Red Lentil Soup with Bacon

Studded with vegetables, this low-fat lentil soup has a light, delicious broth, enhanced by the smoky flavor of low-sodium bacon. Red lentils are used here because of their smaller size and shorter cooking time. If standard brown lentils are used, increase simmering time to 40 minutes.

INGREDIENTS | SERVES 8

2 slices low-sodium bacon, diced

1 medium onion, diced

3 cloves garlic, minced

2 medium carrots, diced

2 medium stalks celery, diced

2 cups dried red lentils, rinsed well

8 cups low-sodium beef broth

2 bay leaves

½ teaspoon dried savory

½ teaspoon dried thyme

¼ teaspoon dried basil

¼ teaspoon dried oregano

⅛ teaspoon dried red pepper flakes

Freshly ground black pepper, to taste

1. Place stockpot over medium heat. Add bacon, onion, and garlic and sauté for 5 minutes.

2. Add carrots and celery and sauté for 2 minutes.

3. Add remaining ingredients and stir well to combine. Raise heat to high and bring to a boil.

4. Once boiling, reduce heat to low, cover pot, and simmer, stirring occasionally, until lentils are tender, 20–30 minutes.

5. Remove from heat, remove bay leaves, and serve.

PER SERVING | Calories: 175 | Fat: 2 g | Protein: 14 g | Sodium: 114 mg | Fiber: 8 g | Carbohydrates: 25 g | Sugar: 3 g

Mushroom Soup with Orzo

A warming dish for a nippy day, this soup is filled with the earthy flavors of mushrooms and garlic.

INGREDIENTS | SERVES 6

24 ounces fresh mushrooms
1 teaspoon olive oil
1 medium onion, diced
1 medium stalk celery, diced
6 cloves garlic, minced
6 cups low-sodium chicken or vegetable broth
½ teaspoon dried rosemary, crumbled
½ teaspoon dried sage, crumbled
½ teaspoon dried thyme
Freshly ground black pepper, to taste
⅔ cup dry orzo pasta

What Is Orzo?

Orzo is a small, oval-shaped pasta, with an appearance similar to rice. It's made from semolina flour, a type of wheat flour, making it an unacceptable choice for those with celiac disease. For a gluten-free alternative, try substituting cooked brown rice.

1. Clean the mushrooms. Slice half of them, chop the rest, and set aside.

2. Heat oil in a stockpot over medium heat. Add the onion, celery, and garlic and sauté for 3 minutes.

3. Add the mushrooms and cook, stirring, for 7 minutes.

4. Add the broth and seasonings, raise heat to high, and bring to a boil.

5. Once boiling, reduce heat to low, add the orzo, and stir well. Cover the pot and simmer 20 minutes.

6. Remove from heat and serve.

PER SERVING | Calories: 138 | Fat: 3 g | Protein: 10 g | Sodium: 75 mg | Fiber: 2 g | Carbohydrates: 21 g | Sugar: 3 g

Sweet Potato and Chickpea Soup

The intoxicating aromas of India were the inspiration for this sensational soup.
Serve hot, garnished with chopped fresh cilantro.

INGREDIENTS | SERVES 4

1 (15-ounce) can no-salt-added garbanzo beans
1 teaspoon olive oil
1 large shallot, chopped
1 garlic clove, minced
1-inch piece fresh ginger, minced
1 teaspoon salt-free garam masala
½ teaspoon ground sweet paprika
⅛ teaspoon dried red pepper flakes
4 cups low-sodium chicken or vegetable broth
4 cups cubed sweet potato
½ cup sliced carrot
2 tablespoons chopped fresh cilantro

1. Drain and rinse the garbanzo beans and set aside.

2. Heat oil in a stockpot over medium heat. Add shallot and garlic and sauté for 2 minutes.

3. Add the ginger and spices and cook, stirring, for 30 seconds.

4. Add the broth and stir to combine. Add the sweet potatoes, carrots, and beans and stir well.

5. Raise heat to high and bring to a boil. Once boiling, cover the pot, reduce heat to medium-low, and simmer for 15 minutes, stirring occasionally.

6. Remove from heat. Ladle into bowls, garnish with fresh cilantro, and serve immediately.

PER SERVING | Calories: 348 | Fat: 5 g | Protein: 16 g | Sodium: 163 mg | Fiber: 10 g | Carbohydrates: 60 g | Sugar: 18 g

Tofu Soup

This low-sodium soup is a natural cure-all. Meaty chunks of tofu and vegetables are bathed in a soft broth with a slightly spicy after-kick.

INGREDIENTS | SERVES 8

8 cups low-sodium vegetable broth
8 cloves garlic, minced
3 medium carrots, diced
4 ounces mushrooms, sliced
4 scallions, sliced
1-inch piece fresh ginger, minced
¼ teaspoon ground white pepper
1 pound extra-firm tofu, cubed
2 scallions, sliced (for garnish)

1. Pour the broth into a stockpot. Add all of the ingredients except for the tofu and last 2 scallions. Bring to a boil over high heat.

2. Once boiling, add the tofu. Reduce heat to low, cover, and simmer for 5 minutes.

3. Remove from heat, ladle soup into bowls, and garnish with the remaining sliced scallions. Serve immediately.

PER SERVING | Calories: 91 | Fat: 3 g | Protein: 6 g | Sodium: 153 mg | Fiber: 2 g | Carbohydrates: 8 g | Sugar: 1 g

Ginger Facts

Ginger, also called gingerroot, has been used for hundreds of years as a natural remedy for many ailments, particularly nausea. It can be eaten raw, cooked, or ground, and adds a spicy, distinctive flavor to both sweet and savory dishes. Ginger contains antioxidants and anti-inflammatory compounds believed to inhibit cancer and cardiovascular disease.

Summer Vegetable Stew

This flavorful dish is light enough for the hottest of days, yet hearty enough to satisfy. Partner with Soft and Crusty No-Rise Bread (Chapter 3) for a lovely meal. Salt-free canned tomatoes may be substituted for fresh when making this out of season.

INGREDIENTS | SERVES 6

2 teaspoons olive oil

1 medium onion, diced

4 cloves garlic, minced

1 small/medium eggplant, peeled and diced

2 small yellow squash, diced

2 small zucchini, diced

6 small tomatoes, diced

2 (8-ounce) cans no-salt-added tomato sauce

1 cup red wine

1 teaspoon dried basil

1 teaspoon dried marjoram

¾ teaspoon freshly ground black pepper

½ teaspoon dried oregano

¼ teaspoon dried savory

1. Heat oil in a sauté pan over medium heat. Add the onion and garlic and sauté for 2 minutes.

2. Add the remaining vegetables and cook, stirring, for 10 minutes.

3. Add remaining ingredients and stir to combine.

4. Cover pot and simmer for 20 minutes, stirring occasionally. Serve warm or at room temperature.

PER SERVING | Calories: 122 | Fat: 2 g | Protein: 2 g | Sodium: 16 mg | Fiber: 3 g | Carbohydrates: 17 g | Sugar: 9 g

Fresh Versus Dried

When adding flavor to uncooked foods such as salads or salsas, fresh herbs are often best. Some herbs, such as parsley and cilantro, don't retain the level of flavor when dried, and their textures suffer, too. When adding herbs to foods that will be cooked or simmered for a length of time, dried herbs may be a better choice. Many dried herbs have a more concentrated flavor than their fresh counterparts and stand up well to cooking. When substituting between the two, use three times the fresh herbs for dried, or 1 tablespoon fresh herb for every 1 teaspoon dried.

Manhattan-Style Seafood Stew

This intoxicating tomato-based stew is filled with the earthy richness of carrots, potatoes, onions, and garlic, the scent of the sea, a touch of citrus, and the kick of cilantro and spicy hot pepper. One bite and you'll agree, it's a salt-free synergy far greater than the sum of its parts. Serve plain or spoon over rice or couscous. Adapted from Prevention's Low-Fat, Low-Cost Freezer Cookbook.

INGREDIENTS | SERVES 6

1½ teaspoons olive oil

1 large onion, diced

4 cloves garlic, minced

2 (15-ounce) cans no-salt-added diced tomatoes

2 medium potatoes, diced

2 cups low-sodium chicken or vegetable broth

2 medium carrots, sliced

½ pound white-fleshed fish, cut into 1-inch chunks

1 jalapeño pepper, minced

1 large bay leaf

¼ pound small shrimp, peeled and cleaned

⅓ cup chopped fresh cilantro

½ teaspoon grated orange zest

½ teaspoon freshly ground black pepper

1. Heat the oil in a small stockpot over medium heat. Add the onion and garlic and cook, stirring, for 3 minutes.

2. Add the tomatoes with juice, potatoes, broth, carrots, fish, minced hot pepper, and bay leaf and stir to combine.

3. Cover the pot and cook, stirring occasionally, for 15 minutes.

4. Add the shrimp, cilantro, orange zest, and black pepper and stir well. Simmer until shrimp are pink, 5 minutes or less, then remove from heat.

5. Carefully remove bay leaf and serve immediately.

PER SERVING | Calories: 163 | Fat: 2 g | Protein: 15 g | Sodium: 169 mg | Fiber: 4 g | Carbohydrates: 22 g | Sugar: 7 g

Chicken, Corn, and Black Bean Chili

This yummy low-sodium chili is a little different from the standard variety, thanks to the addition of corn, meaty chunks of chicken, and the virtual absence of tomatoes. Partner with Perfect Cornbread (Chapter 3) for a truly heavenly meal. Recipe adapted from Kitchen Basics Healthy Cooking with Stock.

INGREDIENTS | SERVES 8

2 (15-ounce) cans no-salt-added black beans

2 teaspoons olive oil

1 pound boneless, skinless chicken breasts, cut into ½-inch cubes

1 medium red onion, diced

3 cloves garlic, minced

1 medium green bell pepper, diced

1 medium red bell pepper, diced

1 (6-ounce) can salt-free tomato paste

2 tablespoons salt-free chili powder

1 teaspoon ground cumin

2 cups low-sodium chicken broth

2 cups frozen corn kernels

¼ cup chopped fresh cilantro

Freshly ground black pepper, to taste

Slow Cooker Magic

Slow cookers take the work out of many meals, and have an almost magical ability to transform the toughest, most inexpensive cuts of meat into tender, succulent feasts. To make this chicken chili in the slow cooker, simply measure ingredients into the appliance, stir to combine, and cover. Set the slow cooker to low and simmer 6–8 hours.

1. Drain and rinse beans and set aside.

2. Heat oil in a large sauté pan over medium heat. Add chicken and sauté until the outside is no longer pink, approximately 3–5 minutes.

3. Add the onion and garlic and sauté for 2 minutes. Add the bell peppers and sauté for 2 minutes.

4. Stir in the tomato paste, chili powder, cumin, broth, and black beans. Raise heat to high and bring to a boil.

5. Once boiling, reduce heat to medium-low, cover, and simmer for 20 minutes.

6. Stir in the corn kernels, cover, and continue cooking for 5 minutes.

7. Remove from heat, stir in the cilantro, and season to taste with freshly ground black pepper. Serve immediately.

PER SERVING | Calories: 309 | Fat: 4 g | Protein: 28 g | Sodium: 81 mg | Fiber: 8 g | Carbohydrates: 42 g | Sugar: 6 g

Two-Bean Tempeh Chili

*A vegan chili everyone will love! Tempeh adds just the right heft,
along with the beans, to make this a year-round crowd pleaser.*

INGREDIENTS | SERVES 8

1 (15-ounce) can no-salt-added kidney beans

1 (15-ounce) can no-salt-added pinto beans

1 (8-ounce) package organic tempeh, cubed

1 medium onion, diced

3 cloves garlic, minced

2 (15-ounce) cans no-salt-added diced tomatoes

2 medium carrots, diced

1 medium bell pepper, diced

1 jalapeño pepper, minced

1 (6-ounce) can salt-free tomato paste

3 (8-ounce) cans no-salt-added tomato sauce

2 teaspoons salt-free chili seasoning

1 teaspoon sugar

1¾ cups frozen corn kernels

¼ cup chopped fresh cilantro

Freshly ground black pepper, to taste

1. Drain and rinse the beans. Set aside.

2. Place a stockpot over medium heat. Add the cubed tempeh, onion, and garlic and sauté for 3 minutes.

3. Add the diced tomatoes, carrot, bell pepper, and jalapeño and sauté for 5 minutes.

4. Stir in the tomato paste, then add the tomato sauce, beans, chili seasoning, and sugar. Stir well to combine. Bring to a boil.

5. Once boiling, reduce heat to low, cover, and simmer for 20 minutes, stirring occasionally.

6. Stir in the corn kernels and simmer just until heated through.

7. Remove pot from heat. Stir in the cilantro and season to taste with black pepper. Serve immediately.

PER SERVING | Calories: 326 | Fat: 4 g | Protein: 19 g | Sodium: 97 mg | Fiber: 12 g | Carbohydrates: 58 g | Sugar: 13 g

CHAPTER 9

Beef

30-Minute Ground Beef Pizza

This supremely delicious pizza is flavored with lean ground beef and fresh veggies.
If you thought "real" pizza was gone from your life, think again!

INGREDIENTS | SERVES 4

1 cup white whole-wheat flour

1 teaspoon all-purpose salt-free seasoning

1 teaspoon salt-free Italian seasoning

½ teaspoon garlic powder

2 egg whites

⅔ cup low-fat milk

½ pound lean ground beef

1 medium onion, chopped

½ cup no-salt-added pasta sauce

2 plum tomatoes, sliced

1 cup sliced mushrooms

1 small bell pepper, diced

3 cloves garlic, minced

¼ cup chopped fresh basil

¼ cup shredded Swiss cheese

¼ cup nonfat ricotta cheese

1. Preheat oven to 425°F. Grease and flour a 12-inch nonstick pizza pan and set aside.

2. Add the flour and seasonings into a mixing bowl and whisk well to combine.

3. Add the egg whites and milk and stir well. Pour batter into the prepared pizza pan and set aside.

4. Place a large skillet over medium heat. Add the ground beef and onion and cook, stirring, for 5 minutes. Remove from heat and carefully drain any excess fat.

5. Spoon mixture evenly over the batter in the pan. Place pan on middle rack in oven and bake for 20 minutes.

6. Once crust is baked, remove pan from oven. Spread pasta sauce evenly over pizza. Top with tomatoes, mushrooms, bell pepper, garlic, chopped basil. Sprinkle the Swiss cheese over the pizza, then dollop with ricotta.

7. Return pan to oven and bake for 5 minutes, until cheese has melted.

8. Remove pizza from oven. Gently remove from pan and cut into 8 slices. Serve immediately.

PER SERVING | Calories: 302 | Fat: 8 g | Protein: 23 g | Sodium: 121 mg | Fiber: 5 g | Carbohydrates: 33 g | Sugar: 6 g

Easy Spaghetti and Meatballs

Who doesn't like spaghetti and meatballs? Here's a simple, delicious, and inexpensive recipe everyone can agree on. As long as you have the ingredients on hand, it's a meal you can whip up anytime. And the meatballs freeze beautifully, too, so feel free to make several batches and stock up for emergencies.

INGREDIENTS | SERVES 8

1 pound extra-lean ground beef
1 medium onion, grated
2 cloves garlic, grated
1 egg white, beaten
½ cup salt-free bread crumbs
1 tablespoon grated Parmesan cheese
1 teaspoon dried basil
½ teaspoon dried oregano
½ teaspoon dried thyme
Freshly ground black pepper, to taste
2 tablespoons olive oil
2 cups no-salt-added pasta sauce
1 pound dry whole-grain spaghetti

Love Spaghetti? Try Spaghetti Squash!

Spaghetti squash is a type of winter squash, with a firm yellow shell and an inner flesh that shreds into pasta-like strands. To cook spaghetti squash, first slice in half lengthwise. Remove the seeds, then place into a microwave-safe bowl. Add ½ cup water, cover, and microwave on high 10–20 minutes, depending upon size. When tender, remove from microwave and shred into strands using a fork.

1. Place ground beef in a mixing bowl and add the grated onion and garlic. Mix together using your (freshly washed) hands.

2. Add the egg white, bread crumbs, cheese, and seasonings, and mix thoroughly.

3. To make the meatballs, pinch off 1–2 tablespoons of the meat mixture and roll between your palms to achieve a nice globe. Set the meatball aside and repeat with remaining meat mixture, until you have roughly 22 (2-inch) meatballs.

4. Heat the olive oil in a large sauté pan over medium heat. Add the meatballs and brown on all sides, roughly 3–5 minutes.

5. Once the meatballs have browned, add the pasta sauce, reduce heat to low, cover, and simmer for 20 minutes, stirring or shaking the pan every so often.

6. Bring a stockpot of water to boil over high heat. Once boiling, add the spaghetti and cook according to directions on the package, omitting salt.

7. Drain, and pour the sauce and meatballs over top. Serve immediately.

PER SERVING | Calories: 387 | Fat: 8 g | Protein: 23 g | Sodium: 63 mg | Fiber: 4 g | Carbohydrates: 54 g | Sugar: 4 g

Whole-Grain Pasta with Meat Sauce

Top your favorite whole-grain pasta with this thick, rich, and hearty salt-free sauce.
If you prefer more spice, increase the amount of crushed red pepper. If not, eliminate it altogether.
Serve with green salad for a complete meal.

INGREDIENTS | SERVES 6

1 pound whole-grain pasta

1 pound extra-lean ground beef

1 medium onion, diced

3 cloves garlic, minced

2 (8-ounce) cans no-salt-added tomato sauce

⅓ cup red wine

1 tablespoon balsamic vinegar

1 teaspoon dried basil

½ teaspoon dried marjoram

½ teaspoon dried oregano

½ teaspoon dried red pepper flakes

½ teaspoon dried thyme

½ teaspoon freshly ground black pepper

1. Cook pasta according to directions on package, omitting salt. Drain and set aside.

2. Place the ground beef, onion, and garlic into a sauté pan over medium heat. Cook, stirring, until beef has browned, about 5 minutes.

3. Add remaining ingredients and stir to combine. Simmer, uncovered, for 10 minutes, stirring occasionally.

4. Remove from heat and spoon over pasta. Serve immediately.

PER SERVING | Calories: 387 | Fat: 5 g | Protein: 27 g | Sodium: 65 mg | Fiber: 9 g | Carbohydrates: 58 g | Sugar: 6 g

Beef Tacos

This mini fiesta will feed 6 people, always a great excuse to have friends over for margaritas. Serve with nonfat sour cream and Holy Guacamole (Chapter 5).

INGREDIENTS | SERVES 6

1 pound extra-lean ground beef

1 large onion, chopped

2 cloves garlic, minced

1 (8-ounce) can no-salt-added tomato sauce

2 teaspoons low-sodium Worcestershire sauce

1 tablespoon molasses

1 tablespoon apple cider vinegar

1 tablespoon ground cumin

1 tablespoon ground sweet paprika

½ teaspoon dried red pepper flakes

Freshly ground black pepper, to taste

1 package low-sodium taco shells

¼ cup chopped fresh cilantro

Low-Sodium Worcestershire Sauce

Traditional Worcestershire sauce derives its unique taste from salted fermented anchovies, and often contains as much as 65 mg of sodium per teaspoon. Fortunately, there are low-sodium versions sold commercially, both in stores and online. Look for either Lea & Perrins or French's Reduced Sodium Worcestershire Sauce.

1. Place the ground beef, onion, and garlic into a sauté pan over medium heat and cook, stirring, until the beef is browned, roughly 3–5 minutes.

2. Once beef is cooked, lower heat to medium-low and add the tomato sauce, Worcestershire sauce, molasses, vinegar, cumin, paprika, red pepper flakes, and black pepper. Simmer, stirring frequently, about 10 minutes.

3. Heat taco shells according to package directions. Remove from oven and set aside.

4. Remove sauté pan from heat. Stir in cilantro, then divide evenly between the taco shells.

5. Garnish with tomato, lettuce, nonfat sour cream, low-sodium salsa, and guacamole, if desired. Serve immediately.

PER SERVING (2 TACOS) | Calories: 255 | Fat: 9 g | Protein: 18 g | Sodium: 79 mg | Fiber: 2 g | Carbohydrates: 23 g | Sugar: 4 g

Dirty Rice

The classic Cajun dish, reworked to be much lower in fat and sodium, but not taste.
This makes a wonderful one-skillet supper or side dish. Adapted from The Healthy Cook.

INGREDIENTS | SERVES 4

½ pound extra-lean ground beef

1 large onion, diced

2 medium stalks celery, diced

2 cloves garlic, minced

1 medium bell pepper, diced

1 teaspoon sodium-free beef bouillon granules

1 cup water

2 teaspoons low-sodium Worcestershire sauce

1½ teaspoons dried thyme

1 teaspoon dried basil

½ teaspoon dried marjoram

¼ teaspoon freshly ground black pepper

Pinch ground cayenne pepper

2 scallions, sliced

3 cups cooked long-grain brown rice

1. Place the ground beef, onion, celery, and garlic into a sauté pan over medium heat. Cook until the beef is browned, roughly 3–5 minutes.

2. Add bell pepper, beef bouillon, water, Worcestershire sauce, and herbs and stir to combine.

3. Bring to a boil, then reduce heat to low, cover, and simmer for 20 minutes.

4. Stir in the scallions and simmer, uncovered, for 3 minutes.

5. Remove from heat. Add the cooked rice and stir well to combine. Serve immediately.

PER SERVING | Calories: 272 | Fat: 4 g | Protein: 16 g | Sodium: 92 mg | Fiber: 4 g | Carbohydrates: 41 g | Sugar: 4 g

Beef with Bok Choy

Bok choy is a small, crunchy Chinese cabbage, with green leaves and squat, white celery-like stalks. This recipe combines stir-fried bok choy with leftover grilled steak for a quick and scrumptious meal. Serve with cooked brown rice if desired.

INGREDIENTS | SERVES 4

2 pounds bok choy

2 teaspoons sesame oil

3 cloves garlic, minced

1 tablespoon minced fresh ginger

1 small red onion, sliced thinly

1 teaspoon sodium-free beef bouillon granules

½ teaspoon ground white pepper

½ cup water

½ pound grilled steak, cut into thin slices

Sesame Oil

The strong fragrance and flavor of sesame oil is often used in Asian cooking, and adds a unique nuance to food without additional sodium. Sesame oil contains 14 g of fat per tablespoon, 12 g of which are unsaturated fat, making it an acceptable part of a healthy diet when used in moderation.

1. To prepare the bok choy, break the individual stalks off at the base, discarding the small central core. Wash the stalks and greens well, then pat dry. Trim each stalk at the base, then cut the stalks and greens into 2-inch pieces.

2. Heat the oil in a wok over medium heat. Add the garlic, ginger, and onion and cook, stirring, for 30 seconds.

3. Add the bok choy and stir-fry for 2 minutes. Add the bouillon, pepper, and water, raise the heat to high, and cook, stirring, for 5–6 minutes.

4. Add the steak and heat through. Remove from heat and serve immediately.

PER SERVING | Calories: 195 | Fat: 10 g | Protein: 20 g | Sodium: 132 mg | Fiber: 2 g | Carbohydrates: 5 g | Sugar: 2 g

Beef with Pea Pods

*A beautifully delicious and 100 percent salt-free take on a Chinese classic,
with toothsome beef and crunchy vegetables. Serve with cooked brown rice.*

INGREDIENTS | SERVES 4

¾ pound thin beef steak (e.g., beef shoulder)

1 tablespoon peanut oil

3 scallions, sliced

2 cloves garlic, minced

2 teaspoons minced fresh ginger

4 cups fresh pea pods, trimmed

3 tablespoons Faux Soy Sauce (see Chapter 5)

4 cups cooked brown rice

1. Slice the beef into thin ½" × 3" strips and set aside.

2. Heat the oil in a wok over medium heat. Add the scallions, garlic, and ginger and stir-fry for 30 seconds.

3. Add the sliced beef and stir-fry for 5 minutes, until beef has browned.

4. Add the pea pods and Faux Soy Sauce and stir-fry for 3 minutes.

5. Remove from heat. Spoon over cooked rice and serve immediately.

PER SERVING | Calories: 466 | Fat: 11 g | Protein: 27 g | Sodium: 71 mg | Fiber: 8 g | Carbohydrates: 64 g | Sugar: 12 g

Pressure Cooker Beef Bourguignon

A simple low-sodium take on the traditional French dish. The pressure cooker cuts cooking time by two-thirds, leaving this ready in just 30 minutes! The heavenly smell of simmering beef and onions will have you (and your lucky guests) salivating.

INGREDIENTS | SERVES 6

2 tablespoons unsalted butter

3 large onions, sliced

2 pounds lean beef stew meat, cubed

2 cups water

1½ cups red wine

2 teaspoons sodium-free beef bouillon granules

½ teaspoon dried marjoram

½ teaspoon dried thyme

½ teaspoon freshly ground black pepper

1 pound white mushrooms, sliced thickly

Pressure Cookers

Pressure cookers are amazing tools, especially on a low-sodium diet. Not only do they speed cooking time and allow you to make meals fast, they retain more nutrients and are one of the most environmentally friendly means of cooking. Opt for a stainless steel appliance, which won't pit from acids in lemon juice, vinegar, and the like.

1. Melt the butter in a pressure cooker over medium-high heat. Add the onions and cook, stirring, for 5 minutes.

2. Move onions to the side of the pan, add the cubed beef, and brown on all sides, about 5 minutes.

3. Add the remaining ingredients and stir to combine. Secure the lid on the pressure cooker and set to high. Raise the heat to high and bring contents to a boil. Once you hear sizzling, reduce heat to medium and cook for 20 minutes.

4. Remove from heat. Allow pressure cooker to depressurize naturally, or place under cold running water for about 5 minutes. Serve immediately.

PER SERVING | Calories: 401 | Fat: 19 g | Protein: 34 g | Sodium: 115 mg | Fiber: 2 g | Carbohydrates: 12 g | Sugar: 5 g

Pressure Cooker Harvest Stew

This hearty low-sodium dish is savory and filling, with an appealing subtle sweetness. Although it looks and tastes impressive, it couldn't be easier; just pop everything into the pressure cooker, and 30 minutes later it's done!

INGREDIENTS | SERVES 6

1 tablespoon olive oil

2 pounds lean beef stew meat, cubed

3 medium carrots, sliced into thick rounds

2 medium tart green apples, cut into chunks

1 large onion, diced

1 cup fresh cranberries, washed

4 cloves garlic, minced

2 cups water

2 teaspoons sodium-free beef bouillon granules

⅓ cup unsweetened apple juice

1 teaspoon dried marjoram

½ teaspoon dried savory

½ teaspoon dried thyme

½ teaspoon ground cinnamon

½ teaspoon ground rosemary

¼ teaspoon ground allspice

Freshly ground black pepper, to taste

1. Heat oil in a pressure cooker over medium-high heat. Add beef cubes and brown on all sides, roughly 3–5 minutes.

2. Add remaining ingredients to the pot and stir to combine. Secure lid on the pressure cooker. Once pressurized, reduce heat to medium and cook for 20 minutes.

3. Remove pressure cooker from heat and place in sink under cold running water. Once cooker is depressurized, remove from sink. Serve immediately.

PER SERVING | Calories: 328 | Fat: 13 g | Protein: 35 g | Sodium: 105 mg | Fiber: 3 g | Carbohydrates: 16 g | Sugar: 10 g

Cottage Pie with Sweet Potato Crust

Ground beef and veggies topped with a heavenly crust of mashed sweet potatoes. A pressure cooker leaves the sweet potatoes fork tender in just 5 minutes; boil for 15–20 minutes if you don't have one.

INGREDIENTS | SERVES 6

3 medium–large sweet potatoes

2 tablespoons unsalted butter

2 tablespoons brown sugar

½ teaspoon ground cinnamon

1 pound extra-lean ground beef

1 medium onion, diced

3 cloves garlic, minced

2 medium carrots, diced

2 medium stalks celery, diced

⅓ cup red wine

1 tablespoon salt-free tomato paste

2 teaspoons sodium-free beef bouillon granules

1 teaspoon dried marjoram

½ teaspoon dried thyme

½ teaspoon freshly ground black pepper

½ teaspoon ground mustard

¼ teaspoon ground rosemary

Shepherd's Pie Versus Cottage Pie

Shepherd's pie is a traditional British dish of ground lamb and vegetables baked beneath a mashed potato crust. Any pie resembling this, but made without lamb or mutton, is referred to as a cottage pie. Cottage pie is most often made with ground beef, but can include any type of meat or nonmeat. Vegetarian versions of both pies are often made with lentils, bulgur, or beans.

1. Preheat oven to 425°F. Take out a 2-quart ovenproof casserole and set aside.

2. Measure 1 cup water into the bottom of your pressure cooker. Place sweet potatoes into the steamer basket and place in pot. Secure lid and place over high heat. Once pressurized, reduce heat to medium-high and cook for 5 minutes.

3. Remove from heat and place pan under cold running water until depressurized. Open pot, drain, and mash sweet potatoes well. Add butter, brown sugar, and cinnamon to pot and stir to combine. Set aside.

4. Heat a sauté pan over medium heat. Add the ground beef, onion, and garlic, and cook, stirring, for 5 minutes.

5. Reduce heat to medium, add remaining ingredients and cook, stirring, for 5 minutes. Remove from heat and spoon beef filling into casserole dish.

6. Spoon mashed sweet potato over top and smooth evenly to form a top crust.

7. Place pan on middle rack in oven and bake for 15 minutes. Remove from oven and serve immediately.

PER SERVING | Calories: 236 | Fat: 8 g | Protein: 17 g | Sodium: 83 mg | Fiber: 3 g | Carbohydrates: 23 g | Sugar: 10 g

Seared Sirloin Steaks with Garlicky Greens

Juicy, medium-rare beef accented with tart and tangy kale or Swiss chard. Serve with roasted potatoes and fresh corn for a spectacular meal in a snap. Adapted from Fine Cooking.

INGREDIENTS | SERVES 6

1½ pounds fresh kale or Swiss chard

1½ pounds sirloin steak, 1 inch thick

1 tablespoon fresh rosemary, coarsely chopped

Freshly ground black pepper, to taste

1 tablespoon olive oil

¾ cup dry white wine

4 cloves garlic, minced

2 tablespoons white balsamic vinegar

1 teaspoon sugar

1 teaspoon salt-free prepared mustard

¼ teaspoon freshly ground black pepper

1. Preheat oven to 400°F. Line a sided baking sheet with aluminum foil and set aside.

2. Wash the greens and pat dry. Trim the leafy greens from the stalks, discard the tough stalks, and chop leaves coarsely. Set aside.

3. Trim and cut the steak into 6 portions. Season both sides of the steaks with rosemary and freshly ground black pepper, to taste.

4. Heat 1 tablespoon olive oil in a sauté pan over medium-high heat. Place steaks in the pan and cook until nicely browned, 3–4 minutes per side. Remove from heat and transfer steaks to the prepared baking sheet. Place on middle rack in oven and roast 5 minutes. Remove from oven and set aside.

5. Return the skillet to medium-high heat. Add the wine and cook, scraping up any browned bits from the bottom of the pan, for 3 minutes. Add the garlic, vinegar, sugar, mustard, and pepper and stir to combine.

6. Add the leafy greens and toss well to coat. Cover the pan and cook, stirring once or twice, until tender, about 5 minutes.

7. Transfer the steaks to plates and top with the greens. Serve immediately.

PER SERVING | Calories: 329 | Fat: 14 g | Protein: 33 g | Sodium: 113 mg | Fiber: 2 g | Carbohydrates: 14 g | Sugar: 2 g

CHAPTER 10

Fish and Seafood

Roasted Salmon with Lemon, Mustard, and Dill

Salmon is best without a lot of fanfare. Here it's roasted simply with a delectably tart and tangy dill glaze.

INGREDIENTS | SERVES 4

1 pound salmon
Juice of 1 fresh lemon
2 tablespoons no-salt-added prepared mustard
2 tablespoons chopped fresh dill
Freshly ground black pepper, to taste

1. Preheat oven to 450°F.

2. Slice salmon into 4 equal fillets and arrange in a baking pan.

3. Combine remaining ingredients in a small mixing bowl and brush tops and sides of fillets with mixture. Drizzle any remaining marinade over top of the fillets.

4. Place pan on middle rack in oven and bake for 10–15 minutes, depending upon thickness of fillets. Salmon is done when it flakes easily with a fork.

5. Remove from oven and serve immediately.

PER SERVING | Calories: 163 | Fat: 7 g | Protein: 22 g | Sodium: 50 mg | Fiber: 0 g | Carbohydrates: <1 g | Sugar: 0 g

Baked Tuna Cakes

*A moist and healthy twist on crab cakes, accented with
veggies and a crisp oven-fried crust.*

INGREDIENTS | SERVES 4

2 (5-ounce) cans no-salt-added tuna, in water

1 small carrot, shredded

1 small stalk celery, finely diced

1 shallot, minced

2 cloves garlic, minced

1 egg white

¼ cup salt-free breadcrumbs

2 tablespoons Salt-Free Mayonnaise (see Chapter 5)

½ teaspoon dried dill

½ teaspoon dried thyme

¼ teaspoon ground rosemary

Freshly ground black pepper, to taste

1. Preheat oven to 400°F. Spray a baking sheet lightly with oil and set aside.

2. Drain the tuna and place in a mixing bowl. Add remaining ingredients and stir well to combine.

3. Shape mixture into 4 equal patties and place on the prepared baking sheet.

4. Place baking sheet on middle rack in oven and bake 10 minutes. Remove from oven, gently flip, and bake 5 minutes more. Remove from oven and serve immediately.

PER SERVING | Calories: 163 | Fat: 5 g | Protein: 20 g | Sodium: 66 mg | Fiber: 1 g | Carbohydrates: 8 g | Sugar: 1 g

Cooking Spray

Cut fat from your diet simply by using a cooking spray. Cooking spray is oil in an aerated form; when sprayed it provides a nonstick surface and the amount of oil is so small as to be negligible. Single-use aerosol cans of cooking spray are sold in supermarkets, but the chemicals they contain make them a poor choice for a healthy lifestyle. Refillable oil spray bottles are sold at many stores and online. These can be used indefinitely, are chemical free, and can be filled with your choice of oil.

Ahi Tuna with Grape Tomato Salsa

Fish always makes a fresh, light, and easy main course, and it's naturally very low in sodium! This recipe calls for broiling the tuna, but it also tastes great grilled. When grilling, 2 minutes per side should be more than enough. Tuna will become tough quickly if overcooked, so be careful.

INGREDIENTS | SERVES 4

2 cups grape tomatoes, halved

¼ cup finely diced onion

¼ cup finely diced green bell pepper

1 clove garlic, minced

1 tablespoon apple cider vinegar

1 tablespoon chopped fresh cilantro

½ teaspoon ground cumin

¼ teaspoon ground coriander

¼ teaspoon freshly ground black pepper

⅛ teaspoon dried red pepper flakes

1 pound ahi (yellowfin) tuna, cut into 4 steaks

1 tablespoon olive oil

Freshly ground black pepper, to taste

Yellowfin Tuna

Yellowfin tuna, also known as ahi, live in the warm waters of the equator and can grow as large as 300–400 pounds. Yellowfin tuna is an excellent source of protein, vitamins B_6 and B_{12}, minerals, and omega-3 fatty acids. It's low in sodium, fat, and calories, making it a great choice on the DASH diet.

1. To make the salsa, add the tomatoes, onion, bell pepper, garlic, vinegar, cilantro, cumin, coriander, black pepper, and pepper flakes into a mixing bowl and stir well to combine. Set aside. Salsa can be made ahead and refrigerated until time to cook.

2. To cook the tuna, preheat broiler. Place the tuna steaks on a broiler pan or in a shallow baking dish, brush lightly with olive oil, and sprinkle with freshly ground black pepper, to taste. Place on top rack in oven and broil for 4 minutes.

3. Remove pan from oven, carefully flip steaks, brush with remaining oil, sprinkle additional pepper, to taste, and return to oven. Broil for another 4 minutes.

4. Remove from oven. Plate each steak with ¼ of the tomato salsa. Serve immediately.

PER SERVING | Calories: 174 | Fat: 4 g | Protein: 27 g | Sodium: 48 mg | Fiber: 1 g | Carbohydrates: 4 g | Sugar: 2 g

Tuna Noodle Casserole

Classic American comfort food at its best. This is a great make-ahead meal: assemble in the morning or the night before, cover, refrigerate, then pop into the oven when you're ready to eat. If you can't find Bragg Organic Sea Kelp Delight, substitute your favorite all-purpose salt-free seasoning. Nonfat plain yogurt may be used instead of sour cream.

INGREDIENTS | SERVES 6

1 pound whole-grain yolkless egg noodles

2 teaspoons canola oil

10 ounces fresh mushrooms, sliced

2 medium carrots, diced

2 medium stalks celery, diced

1 medium bell pepper, diced

1 medium onion, diced

4 cloves garlic, minced

2 (6-ounce) cans no-salt-added tuna in water, drained

1 cup nonfat sour cream

½ cup shredded Swiss cheese

1 teaspoon Bragg Organic Sea Kelp Delight Seasoning

½ teaspoon dried herbes de Provence

Freshly ground black pepper, to taste

1. Cook noodles according to package directions, omitting salt. Drain and set aside.

2. Preheat oven to 375°F. Take out a 3-quart baking dish, spray lightly with oil, and set aside.

3. Heat oil in a sauté pan over medium heat. Add mushrooms, carrots, celery, bell pepper, onion, and garlic and cook, stirring, for 5 minutes. Remove from heat.

4. Add the noodles, along with the remaining ingredients, and stir well to combine.

5. Pour mixture into the prepared dish and cover with lid or aluminum foil. Place on middle rack in oven and bake for 25 minutes.

6. Remove from oven and serve immediately.

PER SERVING | Calories: 434 | Fat: 9 g | Protein: 29 g | Sodium: 137 mg | Fiber: 4 g | Carbohydrates: 55 g | Sugar: 4 g

Healthy Fish and Chips

This healthy, salt-free version of the beloved coastal dinner is baked rather than fried. Choose your favorite white-fleshed fish, such as haddock, pollock, or cod. Serve with lemon wedges, malt vinegar, and salt-free ketchup. Adapted from Let's Cook!

INGREDIENTS | SERVES 4

2 tablespoons unbleached all-purpose flour

2 tablespoons white whole-wheat flour

Freshly ground black pepper, to taste

2 egg whites

2 cups salt-free bread crumbs or panko

1 tablespoon dried herbs (a single herb or mix of favorites, such as parsley, dill, thyme, etc.)

1 pound white-fleshed fish cut into 4 fillets

4 large potatoes, scrubbed

3 tablespoons olive oil

Freshly ground black pepper, to taste

Low-Sodium Tartar Sauce

Whip up a batch of low-sodium tartar sauce in minutes by combining ¼ cup Salt-Free Mayonnaise (see Chapter 5) with a tablespoon of salt-free pickle relish. Use immediately or cover and refrigerate until serving. Salt-free pickle relish is sold at select stores and online.

1. Preheat oven to 425°F. Cover a large baking sheet with foil and set aside.

2. Measure the flours into a wide shallow bowl, add black pepper, and whisk to combine.

3. Place the egg whites into a second shallow bowl.

4. Place bread crumbs in a large plastic bag. Add herbs, seal bag, and shake well.

5. Cut the fish fillets in half, yielding 8 pieces total. Dredge each fillet completely in the seasoned flour, then dip in egg, coating completely.

6. Place the moistened fillet into the plastic bag, seal, and shake gently to coat. Once the fillet is totally coated, carefully remove from bag and place on the baking sheet. Repeat process until all pieces are battered. Place the tray of fish in the refrigerator.

7. Place a piece of parchment on a baking sheet. Cut each potato into 8 equal wedges. Arrange the wedges on the baking sheet and brush both sides lightly with oil. Season, to taste, with freshly ground black pepper.

8. Place baking sheet on the middle rack in the oven and bake for 15 minutes. Remove from oven and flip potatoes over. Return to middle rack in oven.

9. Remove the fish from the fridge and place on the top rack in the oven. Bake potatoes and fish for 15 minutes, until both are crispy and brown. Remove from oven and serve immediately.

PER SERVING | Calories: 534 | Fat: 13 g | Protein: 38 g | Sodium: 142 mg | Fiber: 5 g | Carbohydrates: 65 g | Sugar: 5 g

Roasted Steelhead Trout with Grapefruit Sauce

The fish is roasted simply, just a brush of olive oil and dusting of black pepper is all it takes to make it melt in your mouth. But the sauce elevates it to stardom. The combination of citrus tang, sweetness, and spice is stupendous. So much flavor, and it's salt free! Adapted from Fine Cooking.

INGREDIENTS | SERVES 4

1 pound steelhead trout

3 teaspoons olive oil, divided

Freshly ground black pepper, to taste

2 medium ruby red grapefruits

1 shallot, minced

1 clove garlic, minced

1 teaspoon minced fresh ginger

2 teaspoons agave nectar

⅛ teaspoon ground cayenne pepper

2 tablespoons thinly sliced fresh basil

1. Preheat the oven to 350°F. Place the steelhead trout in a baking dish, brush with 2 teaspoons olive oil, and season with freshly ground black pepper to taste. Place the pan on the middle rack in the oven and roast for 15 minutes.

2. To prepare the sauce, cut the top and bottom off one of the grapefruits. Stand on one end and cut down to remove the white pith and peel. Use a sharp knife to remove each grapefruit segment from its membrane. Cut the segments in half and set aside. Juice the other grapefruit and set aside.

3. Heat the remaining teaspoon of olive oil in a saucepan over medium heat. Add the shallot and garlic and sauté for 2 minutes.

4. Add the ginger, grapefruit juice, agave nectar, and cayenne and stir to combine. Bring to a simmer, then cook until reduced by half, about 10 minutes.

5. Remove saucepan from heat. Stir in the grapefruit and basil.

6. Remove trout from oven. Slice into 4 portions, garnish with sauce, and serve immediately.

PER SERVING | Calories: 250 | Fat: 7 g | Protein: 24 g | Sodium: 36 mg | Fiber: 2 g | Carbohydrates: 22 g | Sugar: 16 g

Southwestern Salmon

Broiled salmon with a kick. The colorful seasoning mix is as pretty as it is flavorful, and the resulting fish is crisp, juicy, and delicious. Pair with Southwestern Rice Pilaf (Chapter 15) for a spectacular salt-free meal.

INGREDIENTS | SERVES 4

1 teaspoon dried cilantro

1 teaspoon ground cumin

1 teaspoon ground paprika

½ teaspoon freshly ground black pepper

½ teaspoon ground coriander

⅛ teaspoon ground cayenne pepper

1 pound boneless salmon fillet

Savory Broiled Salmon

Combine 1 teaspoon dried marjoram, ½ teaspoon each dried savory and ground white pepper, and ¼ teaspoon each dried thyme, ground rosemary, and garlic powder in a small bowl. Rub the mixture into a 1-pound boneless salmon fillet, then broil 7–8 minutes. The rub adds an extra jolt of flavor to an already tasty fish, and the broiling process renders the flesh crisp outside and juicy within.

1. Preheat broiler and move a rack to the top of the oven. Spray a baking sheet lightly with oil and set aside.

2. Place the seasonings into a small bowl and mix well to combine.

3. Sprinkle the spice mixture over the salmon fillet and gently rub the mixture into the fish. Place the fillet in the prepared pan.

4. Place the pan on the top rack in the oven and broil for about 7 minutes, 1–2 minutes less for thin fillets, a little longer for thicker fillets. When cooked fully, salmon will be opaque and flake easily.

5. Remove pan from oven, slice salmon into 4 portions, and serve immediately.

PER SERVING | Calories: 171 | Fat: 8 g | Protein: 22 g | Sodium: 50 mg | Fiber: 0 g | Carbohydrates: 0 g | Sugar: 0 g

Spicy Tilapia with Pineapple Relish

Tilapia is a terrific fish—mild in flavor, meaty, and often inexpensive. This recipe calls for salt-free Cajun seasoning. If you don't have any on hand, try Benson's Salt Free Calypso or Mrs. Dash Caribbean Citrus. For those with an aversion to spicy food, omit the red pepper flakes and jalapeño. Adapted from Cooking Light.

INGREDIENTS | SERVES 4

½ medium pineapple, diced

1 small red onion, diced

1 small tomato, diced

1 jalapeño pepper, minced

2 cloves garlic, minced

2 tablespoons plain unflavored rice vinegar

2 tablespoons chopped fresh cilantro

2 teaspoons canola oil

1 teaspoon salt-free Cajun seasoning

¼ teaspoon dried red pepper flakes

1 pound boneless tilapia fillet

1. Combine pineapple, onion, tomato, jalapeño, and garlic in a mixing bowl. Add the vinegar and cilantro and stir to combine.

2. Heat oil in a large sauté pan over medium-high heat.

3. Combine Cajun seasoning and red pepper flakes in a small bowl and sprinkle evenly over the fish. Place fish in pan and cook for 2 minutes per side, or until fish flakes easily when tested with a fork.

4. Remove from heat and serve immediately, dividing the fish into 4 portions and plating each with a quarter of the pineapple relish.

PER SERVING | Calories: 220 | Fat: 4 g | Protein: 24 g | Sodium: 68 mg | Fiber: 2 g | Carbohydrates: 22 g | Sugar: 16 g

Shrimp Creole

Amazing flavor with none of the salt! This spicy and beautiful shrimp dish is made for special occasions. Serve over cooked brown or white rice.

INGREDIENTS | SERVES 6

2 teaspoons canola oil

1 medium onion, thinly sliced

1 medium bell pepper, thinly sliced

2 medium stalks celery, thinly sliced

3 cloves garlic, minced

2 (15-ounce) cans no-salt-added diced tomatoes

1 (8-ounce) can no-salt-added tomato sauce

⅓ cup white wine

½ teaspoon apple cider vinegar

2 bay leaves

2 teaspoons salt-free chili seasoning

1 teaspoon ground sweet paprika

½ teaspoon freshly ground black pepper

⅛ teaspoon ground cayenne pepper

1 pound peeled shrimp, tails removed

1. Heat oil in a sauté pan over medium heat. Add the onion, bell pepper, celery, and garlic and cook, stirring, for 5 minutes.

2. Add the remaining ingredients except shrimp and stir well to combine. Simmer for 10 minutes, stirring frequently. Cover and reduce heat to medium-low if sauce begins to splatter.

3. Stir in the shrimp and simmer for 5 minutes.

4. Remove from heat and remove bay leaves from pan. Serve immediately.

PER SERVING | Calories: 152 | Fat: 3 g | Protein: 17 g | Sodium: 136 mg | Fiber: 2 g | Carbohydrates: 11 g | Sugar: 6 g

The Skinny on Shrimp

Shrimp are fairly high in sodium naturally, at roughly 160 mg per 3 ounce serving, so they should be consumed carefully. Shrimp come in a variety of sizes, from miniscule to extra colossal, and are typically sold by weight and size; for instance, a pound of large shrimp contains roughly 30–35 pieces. Most shrimp consumed in the United States have been processed to some degree and may have added salt. Read package labels carefully and buy fresh, unprocessed shrimp whenever possible.

Barbecue Pizza with Ground Pork, Peppers, and Pineapple

So much flavor, you won't believe it's salt free! Check Chapter 5 for a delicious sauce (Spicy, Sweet, and Tangy Barbecue Sauce) perfect for this pizza.

INGREDIENTS | SERVES 4

1 cup white whole-wheat flour

1 teaspoon all-purpose salt-free seasoning

1 teaspoon salt-free Italian seasoning

½ teaspoon garlic powder

2 egg whites

⅔ cup low-fat milk

½ pound lean ground pork

2 teaspoons salt-free chili seasoning

1 medium red onion, chopped

½ cup Spicy, Sweet, and Tangy Barbecue Sauce (see Chapter 5), or equivalent

1 cup diced fresh pineapple

1 small red bell pepper, diced

1 jalapeño pepper, minced

3 cloves garlic, minced

2 tablespoons chopped fresh cilantro

¼ cup shredded Swiss cheese

1. Preheat oven to 425°F. Grease and flour a 12-inch nonstick pizza pan and set aside.

2. Place the flour and seasonings into a mixing bowl and whisk well to combine.

3. Add the egg whites and milk and stir well. Pour batter into the prepared pizza pan and set aside.

4. Place a large skillet over medium heat. Add the ground pork, salt-free chili seasoning, and onion and cook, stirring, for 5 minutes. Remove from heat and carefully drain any excess fat.

5. Spoon mixture evenly over the batter in the pan. Place pan on middle rack in oven and bake for 20 minutes.

6. Spread barbecue sauce evenly over pizza, then top with pineapple, peppers, garlic, and chopped cilantro. Sprinkle the Swiss cheese over the pizza.

7. Return pan to oven and bake for 3–5 minutes, until cheese has melted.

8. Remove pizza from oven. Gently remove from pan and cut into 8 slices. Serve immediately.

PER SERVING | Calories: 306 | Fat: 7 g | Protein: 21 g | Sodium: 98 mg | Fiber: 5 g | Carbohydrates: 39 g | Sugar: 12 g

Asian-Inspired Mini Meatloaves with Salt-Free Hoisin Glaze

*Deliciously meaty, these seductive little loaves are loaded with veggies and
the mingling flavors of ginger, garlic, and 5-spice powder.*

INGREDIENTS | SERVES 4

½ pound lean ground pork
1 medium red bell pepper, diced
¾ cup shelled edamame
3 scallions, sliced
3 cloves garlic, minced
1 tablespoon minced fresh ginger
1 egg white
⅓ cup salt-free bread crumbs
½ teaspoon ground 5-spice powder
¼ teaspoon ground white pepper
3 tablespoons Faux Soy Sauce, divided
(see Chapter 5)
1 tablespoon salt-free tomato paste

Salt-Free Hoisin Sauce

To make a delicious salt-free hoisin sauce,
combine 2 parts Faux Soy Sauce (see
Chapter 5) and 1 part salt-free tomato
paste, and stir until smooth. Use immediately or store in an airtight container and
refrigerate until needed.

1. Preheat oven to 375°F. Spray 4 cups of a jumbo muffin tin lightly with oil and set aside.

2. Place the pork, bell pepper, edamame, scallions, garlic, ginger, egg white, bread crumbs, 5-spice powder, and pepper into a bowl. Add 1 tablespoon Faux Soy Sauce and mix together using your (freshly washed) hands.

3. Divide mixture into 4 equal portions and press into the prepared muffin tin.

4. Measure the remaining 2 tablespoons Faux Soy Sauce and tomato paste into a small bowl and stir until smooth. Brush onto the tops of the meatloaves, dividing evenly.

5. Place muffin tin on middle rack in oven and bake for 30 minutes.

6. Remove from oven, gently run a knife around the sides of each loaf, and remove from tin. Serve immediately.

PER SERVING | Calories: 205 | Fat: 6 g | Protein: 17 g |
Sodium: 56 mg | Fiber: 3 g | Carbohydrates: 20 g | Sugar: 7 g

Whole-Grain Rotini with Pork, Pumpkin, and Sage

A deliciously filling main dish. The pumpkin adds color, nutrients, and subtle flavor.
Rotini, corkscrew-shaped pasta with a lot of surface area, allows the sauce to really cling.
Feel free to substitute a different variety of pasta if you prefer.

INGREDIENTS | SERVES 6

1 (13-ounce) package whole-grain rotini
1 pound lean ground pork
1 medium red onion, diced
3 cloves garlic, minced
1 medium bell pepper, diced
1 cup pumpkin purée
2 teaspoons ground sage
1 teaspoon ground rosemary
½–1 teaspoon freshly ground black pepper, to taste

1. Cook pasta according to package directions, omitting salt. Drain and set aside.

2. Heat sauté pan over medium heat. Add ground pork, onion, and garlic and sauté for 2 minutes.

3. Add bell pepper and sauté for 5 minutes.

4. Remove from heat. Add pasta to pan along with remaining ingredients. Stir well to combine. Serve immediately.

PER SERVING | Calories: 331 | Fat: 7 g | Protein: 23 g | Sodium: 48 mg | Fiber: 8 g | Carbohydrates: 45 g | Sugar: 3 g

Pork Chops with Sautéed Apples and Shallots

Fill your house with the heavenly smell of apples and cinnamon.
These boneless medallions in a white wine sauce are 100 percent salt free and delicious.

INGREDIENTS | SERVES 4

1 pound pork loin chops
Freshly ground black pepper, to taste
1 teaspoon olive oil
3 shallots, minced, divided
¾ cup white wine
Freshly ground black pepper, to taste
2 tablespoons unsalted butter
4 medium apples, sliced thinly
½ cup apple juice
¼ cup brown sugar
½ teaspoon ground cinnamon

Pork Facts

Lean pork is considered a healthy meat, containing roughly the same cholesterol per serving as chicken and turkey. It is an excellent source of protein, vitamins B_6 and B_{12}, and minerals. Its mild flavor is a great partner to most types of fruit, both fresh and dried. As a lean meat, pork can dry out quickly, so it's important not to overcook.

1. Preheat oven to 350°F. Take out a baking dish and set aside.

2. Season chops with black pepper. Heat oil in a sauté pan over medium-high heat. Place chops in pan and brown quickly on both sides, roughly 2–3 minutes. Remove from pan and transfer to baking dish.

3. Reduce heat to medium. Add 2 of the minced shallots to pan and cook, stirring, for 2–3 minutes, scraping pan to remove drippings.

4. Add wine and black pepper, to taste. Cook, stirring, for 1 minute, then pour over chops.

5. Cover baking dish with aluminum foil, place on middle rack in oven, and bake for 30 minutes, until internal temperature reaches 145°F.

6. To prepare the apples, melt butter in a sauté pan over medium heat. Add the remaining minced shallot and sauté for 2 minutes.

7. Add remaining ingredients and cook, stirring, for 10–15 minutes, until apples are tender.

8. Remove pan from heat. Remove pork chops from oven. Plate each chop with ¼ of the sautéed apples and shallots. Serve immediately.

PER SERVING | Calories: 396 | Fat: 11 g | Protein: 28 g | Sodium: 277 mg | Fiber: 2 g | Carbohydrates: 40 g | Sugar: 32 g

Ginger and Garlic Pork Stir-Fry

Intensely flavorful and speedy to prepare, this low-sodium stir-fry features tender pork loin and crisp veggies in a delectable sauce. Serve over cooked brown rice.

INGREDIENTS | SERVES 4

8 ounces pork tenderloin, sliced thinly

1½ tablespoons minced fresh ginger

3 cloves garlic, minced

2 tablespoons Faux Soy Sauce (see Chapter 5)

¾ cup low-sodium vegetable broth

2 teaspoons cornstarch

2 teaspoons sesame oil

1 head bok choy, sliced

½ pound pea pods or sugar snap peas

2 medium carrots, sliced

1 medium red bell pepper, diced

1 small red onion, diced

4 scallions, sliced

Freshly ground black pepper, to taste

1. Place pork into a mixing bowl, add the minced ginger, garlic, and Faux Soy Sauce and stir well to coat. Set aside.

2. Measure the broth and cornstarch into a second bowl and whisk well to combine. Set aside.

3. Heat the oil in a wok over medium heat. Add the bok choy, pea pods, carrots, bell pepper, and onion and cook, stirring, for 5 minutes.

4. Add the pork mixture and cook, stirring, for 3 minutes.

5. Add the broth mixture and cook, stirring, until sauce thickens, roughly 30 seconds to 1 minute.

6. Remove from heat. Stir in the sliced scallions and season with freshly ground black pepper to taste. Serve immediately.

PER SERVING | Calories: 180 | Fat: 4 g | Protein: 17 g | Sodium: 323 mg | Fiber: 5 g | Carbohydrates: 20 g | Sugar: 10 g

30-Minute Lamb Pizza with Pine Nuts, Sundried Tomatoes, and Ricotta

An intensely flavorful yet low in sodium pizza.
Sundried tomatoes add tremendous depth; opt for those without oil.

INGREDIENTS | SERVES 4

1 cup white whole-wheat flour

1 teaspoon all-purpose salt-free seasoning

1 teaspoon salt-free Italian seasoning

½ teaspoon garlic powder

2 egg whites

⅔ cup low-fat milk

½ pound lean ground lamb

1 medium onion, chopped

1 medium apple, cored and chopped

¼ cup sundried tomatoes or sliced plum tomatoes

2 tablespoons pine nuts

2 cloves garlic, thinly sliced

2 tablespoons chopped fresh mint

¼ cup Swiss cheese, shredded

¼ cup nonfat ricotta cheese

Freshly ground black pepper, to taste

Pine Nuts

Pine nuts are the edible seeds of several species of pine trees and are often associated with Italian, Greek, and other cuisines. Pine nuts can be expensive, but the distinctive flavor they add to dishes, especially homemade pesto, is priceless. Store pine nuts in the refrigerator to preserve their taste and texture.

1. Preheat oven to 425°F. Grease and flour a 12-inch nonstick pizza pan and set aside.

2. Measure the flour and seasonings into a mixing bowl and whisk well to combine.

3. Add the egg whites and milk and stir well. Pour batter into the prepared pizza pan and set aside.

4. Place a large skillet over medium heat. Add the ground lamb and onion and cook, stirring, for 5 minutes.

5. Remove from heat and carefully drain any excess fat. Spoon mixture evenly over the batter in the pan. Place pan on middle rack in oven and bake for 20 minutes.

6. Once crust is baked, remove pan from oven. Top pizza with apple, tomatoes, pine nuts, garlic, and mint. Sprinkle the Swiss cheese over the pizza, then dollop with the ricotta. Season with freshly ground black pepper, to taste.

7. Return pan to oven and bake for 3–5 minutes, until cheese has melted.

8. Remove pizza from oven. Gently remove from pan and cut into 8 slices. Serve immediately.

PER SERVING | Calories: 220 | Fat: 9 g | Protein: 13 g | Sodium: 114 mg | Fiber: 3 g | Carbohydrates: 22 g | Sugar: 6 g

Mini Shepherd's Pies

Ground lamb and veggies in a flavorful sauce,
beneath a crisp blanket of mashed potatoes.

INGREDIENTS | SERVES 4

3 cups diced potato

½ pound lean ground lamb

1 small onion, diced

3 cloves garlic, minced

1 medium carrot, diced

1 medium stalk celery, diced

1 cup frozen peas

2 tablespoons no-salt-added tomato paste

1 teaspoon dried oregano

½ teaspoon dried basil

½ teaspoon dried thyme

¼ teaspoon freshly ground black pepper

5 tablespoons low-fat milk

2 tablespoons nonfat sour cream

1 tablespoon unsalted butter

1 teaspoon all-purpose salt-free seasoning

1 teaspoon onion powder

½ teaspoon garlic powder

Freshly ground black pepper, to taste

1. Preheat oven to 450°F. Take out 4 (4-inch) ramekins and set aside.

2. Place diced potato in a saucepan and add enough water to cover by 1 inch. Bring to a boil over high heat, then reduce heat to medium and continue boiling for 10 minutes.

3. While the potatoes are boiling, heat a large skillet over medium-high heat. Add lamb, onion, garlic, carrot, and celery and cook, stirring, for 5 minutes.

4. In the last minute of cooking, stir in the peas, tomato paste, and herbs. Spoon contents into the ramekins.

5. Once the potatoes are tender, drain, then mash. Add the remaining ingredients and stir well to combine.

6. Spoon ¼ of the mashed potato mixture into each ramekin and smooth, making sure edges are completely sealed. Place ramekins on a baking sheet. Place sheet on middle rack in oven and bake for 10 minutes.

7. Remove from oven and serve immediately.

PER SERVING | Calories: 294 | Fat: 13 g | Protein: 15 g | Sodium: 89 mg | Fiber: 4 g | Carbohydrates: 30 g | Sugar: 6 g

Lamb Curry with Tomatoes and Spinach

Simple yet substantial, this curry of lamb and vegetables in a savory sauce comes together in mere minutes. If you like spice, add a minced hot pepper or a pinch of ground cayenne at the end of cooking. Serve over brown or white basmati rice.

INGREDIENTS | SERVES 4

1 teaspoon olive oil

1 pound lean boneless lamb, sliced thinly

1 large onion, diced

3 cloves garlic, minced

1 medium red bell pepper, diced

2 tablespoons salt-free tomato paste

1 tablespoon salt-free curry powder

1 (15-ounce) can no-salt-added diced tomatoes

10 ounces fresh baby spinach

½ cup low-sodium beef or vegetable broth

¼ cup red wine

¼ cup chopped fresh cilantro

Freshly ground black pepper, to taste

1. Heat the oil in a sauté pan over medium heat. Add the lamb and brown on both sides, about 2 minutes.

2. Add the onion, garlic, and bell pepper and cook, stirring, for 2 minutes. Stir in the tomato paste and curry powder.

3. Add the tomatoes with juice, spinach, broth, and wine and stir well to combine, scraping up any brown bits from the bottom of the pan. Cook, stirring, until spinach has wilted and lamb has cooked through, about 3–4 minutes.

4. Remove from heat. Stir in the cilantro and season to taste with black pepper. Serve immediately.

PER SERVING | Calories: 238 | Fat: 7 g | Protein: 27 g | Sodium: 167 mg | Fiber: 4 g | Carbohydrates: 14 g | Sugar: 6 g

Lamb Meatballs with Whole-Grain Couscous

These fragrant meatballs make a nice change of pace from traditional beef, and taste equally great spooned over cooked pasta or rice. Serve with green salad or veggies for a complete meal.

INGREDIENTS | SERVES 4

1½ cups water
1 cup whole-wheat couscous
1 pound lean ground lamb
¼ cup pine nuts or walnuts, chopped
1 medium red onion, chopped finely
3 cloves garlic, minced
1 egg white
½ cup salt-free bread crumbs
¼ cup chopped fresh parsley
1 tablespoon chopped fresh mint
Freshly ground black pepper, to taste
1 teaspoon olive oil
2 (8-ounce) cans no-salt-added tomato sauce
2 tablespoons salt-free tomato paste
¼ cup red wine
1 teaspoon dried basil
½ teaspoon dried marjoram
¼ teaspoon dried thyme

Lamb Facts

Lean lamb is a low-sodium food, containing on average less than 70 mg sodium per serving. It's high in protein, an excellent source of B vitamins and minerals, and low in calories and cholesterol. Lamb can be prepared in the same ways as other red meats—grilled, broiled, baked, or pan fried. Its distinct taste marries well with strong flavors such as garlic, mustard, rosemary, curry, and wine.

1. Measure water into a saucepan and bring to a boil over high heat.

2. Once boiling, stir in the couscous, reduce heat to medium-low, cover, and simmer for 2 minutes. Remove pot from heat, remove lid, and fluff couscous with a fork. Let stand for 5 minutes.

3. Place the ground lamb, pine nuts, onion, garlic, egg white, bread crumbs, parsley, and mint into a mixing bowl. Season with black pepper to taste. Mix together using your (freshly washed) hands and form into 2-inch meatballs.

4. Heat the oil in a sauté pan over medium heat. Add meatballs and brown on all sides, roughly 3–5 minutes. Briefly remove from heat.

5. Place the tomato sauce, tomato paste, wine, and seasonings into a mixing bowl and whisk well to combine. Pour mixture over the meatballs and gently stir.

6. Return sauté pan to heat. Once the sauce begins to boil, reduce heat to medium-low, cover, and simmer until meatballs are cooked through, about 15–20 minutes, stirring frequently.

7. Remove from heat and spoon over cooked couscous. Serve immediately.

PER SERVING | Calories: 630 | Fat: 28 g | Protein: 32 g | Sodium: 129 mg | Fiber: 6 g | Carbohydrates: 62 g | Sugar: 13 g

CHAPTER 12

Poultry

Broccoli, Ground Turkey, and Pesto Pizza

Lean ground turkey, savory red onion, broccoli, and pesto make this a low-sodium pizza you won't forget. And it's ready in just 30 minutes!

INGREDIENTS | SERVES 4

1 cup white whole-wheat flour

1 teaspoon all-purpose salt-free seasoning

1 teaspoon salt-free Italian seasoning

½ teaspoon garlic powder

2 egg whites

⅔ cup low-fat milk

½ pound lean ground turkey

1 medium red onion, chopped

1 teaspoon olive oil

1 medium red bell pepper, diced

1 head broccoli, chopped

4 tablespoons Basil Pesto (see Chapter 5)

½ cup Swiss cheese, shredded

Freshly ground black pepper, to taste

1. Preheat oven to 425°F. Grease and flour a 12-inch nonstick pizza pan and set aside.

2. Place the flour and seasonings into a mixing bowl and whisk well to combine. Add the egg whites and milk and stir well. Pour batter into the prepared pizza pan and set aside.

3. Place a large skillet over medium heat. Add the ground turkey and onion and cook, stirring, for 5 minutes.

4. Remove from heat and carefully drain any excess fat. Spoon mixture evenly over the batter in the pan. Place pan on middle rack in oven and bake for 20 minutes.

5. While pizza is baking, heat oil in a sauté pan over medium heat. Add the bell pepper and broccoli and sauté for 5 minutes. Remove pan from heat and set aside.

6. Once crust is baked, remove pan from oven. Top pizza with pesto, spreading evenly. Arrange broccoli and peppers evenly over top, then sprinkle with Swiss cheese and freshly ground black pepper, to taste. Return pan to oven and bake for 3–5 minutes, until cheese has melted completely.

7. Remove pizza from oven. Gently remove from pan and cut into 8 slices. Serve immediately.

PER SERVING | Calories: 327 | Fat: 14 g | Protein: 22 g | Sodium: 131 mg | Fiber: 5 g | Carbohydrates: 30 g | Sugar: 4 g

Ground Turkey Meatloaf Minis

A deliciously lighter version of the all-American meal, these mini meatloaves can also be made with lean ground chicken. Serve with Garlic Rosemary Mashed Potatoes (see Chapter 15).

INGREDIENTS | SERVES 6

1½ pounds lean ground turkey
1 medium onion, finely diced
2 medium stalks celery, finely diced
1 small bell pepper, finely diced
4 cloves garlic, minced
1 (8-ounce) can no-salt-added tomato sauce
1 egg white
¾ cup salt-free bread crumbs
1 tablespoon molasses
¼ teaspoon liquid smoke
½ teaspoon dried basil
½ teaspoon dried oregano
½ teaspoon dried savory
½ teaspoon dried thyme
½ teaspoon freshly ground black pepper
¼ cup salt-free ketchup

1. Preheat oven to 375°F. Spray a 6-cup jumbo muffin tin lightly with oil and set aside.

2. Place all of the ingredients except ketchup into a large bowl and mix well using your (freshly washed) hands.

3. Divide mixture evenly between the muffin cups and press in firmly.

4. Divide the ketchup between the muffin cups and spread evenly for a nice glaze.

5. Place muffin tin on middle rack in oven and bake for 30 minutes.

6. Remove from oven. Gently run a knife around the sides of each loaf and remove from tin. Serve immediately.

PER SERVING | Calories: 251 | Fat: 7 g | Protein: 25 g | Sodium: 112 mg | Fiber: 2 g | Carbohydrates: 21 g | Sugar: 7 g

Homemade Bread Crumbs

To make your own salt-free bread crumbs, crisp several pieces of salt-free or low-sodium bread in the toaster or conventional oven. Tear or crumb the toasted bread into tiny pieces; for a fine crumb, pulse in a food processor. Wonderful low-sodium bread crumbs can also be made from finely chopped unsalted nuts, matzo, and salt-free potato chips.

Turkey and Brown Rice Stuffed Peppers

There are as many ways to stuff a pepper as there are stars in the sky. This version uses ground turkey and brown rice, with juicy tomatoes and raisins for a little added sweetness.

INGREDIENTS | SERVES 4

4 large bell peppers
1 pound lean ground turkey
1 medium onion, diced
3 cloves garlic, minced
2 medium stalks celery, diced
2 cups cooked brown rice
1 (15-ounce) can no-salt-added diced tomatoes
2 tablespoons salt-free tomato paste
¼ cup seedless raisins
2 teaspoons ground cumin
1 teaspoon dried oregano
½ teaspoon ground cinnamon
½ teaspoon freshly ground black pepper

1. Preheat the oven to 425°F. Lightly spray a 9" × 13" baking pan with oil and set aside.

2. Wash and dry the peppers. Trim about ½ inch off the top and place caps aside. Carefully core and seed, leaving the peppers intact. Trim bottoms if necessary so that the peppers sit flat. Set aside.

3. Heat a sauté pan over medium heat. Add the ground turkey, onion, garlic, and celery and sauté for 5 minutes. Remove from heat.

4. Stir in the remaining ingredients and mix well.

5. Fill each pepper with ¼ of the mixture, pressing firmly to pack. Stand peppers in the prepared baking pan, replace the pepper caps, and then cover pan tightly with foil. Place pan on middle rack in oven and bake until tender, about 25–30 minutes.

6. Remove from oven and serve immediately.

PER SERVING | Calories: 354 | Fat: 8 g | Protein: 27 g | Sodium: 126 mg | Fiber: 6 g | Carbohydrates: 45 g | Sugar: 14 g

Lemon Thyme Turkey Meatballs

Juicy inside with a meaty outer crust, each bite of these meatballs is heightened with citrus and the heavenly scent of thyme. Serve over whole-grain noodles. Adapted from Eating Well Magazine.

INGREDIENTS | SERVES 6

¼ cup white whole-wheat flour

1 medium onion, cut into chunks

3 cloves garlic

Grated zest of 1 fresh lemon

1½ teaspoons dried thyme, divided

1 pound lean ground turkey

¾ cup salt-free bread crumbs

3 tablespoons grated Parmesan cheese

¼ teaspoon freshly ground black pepper

2 teaspoons olive oil

½ cup dry white wine

1¾ cups low-sodium chicken broth

1½ tablespoons freshly squeezed lemon juice

Talking Turkey

Skinless turkey is a lean meat, containing less than 4 g fat per 3-ounce serving. Like chicken, it's high in vitamin B_6, protein, and minerals. Although considered a consummate holiday food, turkey consumption is on the rise in the United States, as companies provide greater diversity of turkey products. Some items, such as turkey bacon and deli meats, are now being offered in low-sodium versions.

1. Place flour into a shallow bowl and set aside.

2. Place onion, garlic, zest, and 1 teaspoon thyme in a food processor and pulse briefly.

3. Transfer mixture to a large bowl and mix in the turkey, crumbs, cheese, and pepper. Pinch off 2 tablespoons at a time and shape into meatballs. Roll the meatballs in the flour to lightly coat. Reserve the remaining flour.

4. Heat oil in a sauté pan over medium heat. Add meatballs and cook, until browned, about 5 minutes. Remove the meatballs from the pan and set aside.

5. Add wine to the pan, increase heat to medium-high, and cook, scraping up any browned bits, until almost evaporated, about 1 minute.

6. Add the broth and bring to a boil. Reduce heat to low and return the meatballs to the pan with the remaining thyme. Cover and cook about 10 minutes.

7. Remove the meatballs again and set aside. Bring the sauce to a boil over medium-high and cook until reduced to about 1 cup, roughly 5 minutes.

8. Add the lemon juice and 1 tablespoon of the flour into a small bowl and whisk until smooth. Add this flour mixture to the sauce and simmer, whisking constantly, until slightly thickened, roughly 1–2 minutes. Remove from heat and add meatballs, swirling to coat. Serve immediately.

PER SERVING | Calories: 226 | Fat: 8 g | Protein: 20 g | Sodium: 117 mg | Fiber: 1 g | Carbohydrates: 17 g | Sugar: 1 g

Grilled Tequila Chicken with Sautéed Peppers and Onion

This fabulous chicken is succulently moist and unbelievably flavorful thanks to the tequila marinade. The longer the chicken steeps, the greater the flavor, so if possible, make the marinade first thing in the morning and let the chicken steep all day. Serve with fresh corn on the cob, nonfat sour cream, and chopped fresh cilantro.

INGREDIENTS | SERVES 4

1 cup lime juice

⅓ cup tequila

3 cloves garlic, chopped

¼ cup chopped fresh cilantro

1 tablespoon agave nectar

½ teaspoon freshly ground black pepper

1 teaspoon cumin

½ teaspoon ground coriander

4 boneless, skinless chicken breasts

2 teaspoons canola oil

1 large green bell pepper, diced

1 large red bell pepper, diced

1 large onion, diced

½ cup nonfat sour cream

1. Add the lime juice, tequila, garlic, cilantro, agave nectar, black pepper, cumin, and coriander into a mixing bowl and whisk well to combine.

2. Add the chicken breasts and turn several times to coat. Cover and refrigerate. Allow to marinate for at least 6 hours, preferably overnight.

3. Heat the grill. Once ready, cook chicken until no longer pink but still juicy and tender, about 10–15 minutes per side.

4. While chicken is grilling, heat the oil in a sauté pan over medium heat. Add the diced peppers and onion and cook, stirring, for 5 minutes. Remove from heat.

5. Remove chicken from grill. Plate each breast with ¼ of the veggies and a dollop of sour cream. Serve immediately.

PER SERVING | Calories: 259 | Fat: 3 g | Protein: 28 g | Sodium: 118 mg | Fiber: 1 g | Carbohydrates: 18 g | Sugar: 7 g

Chicken, Black Bean, and Veggie Soft Tacos

Soft corn tortillas filled with a saucy and spicy combination of chicken, veggies, and beans. If you're using a commercial chili seasoning, start with a teaspoon and work up from there.

INGREDIENTS | SERVES 6

1 package 5-inch corn tortillas
3 boneless, skinless chicken thighs
½ cup low-sodium chicken broth
1 medium carrot, diced
1 medium sweet potato, diced
1 medium onion, diced
1 medium bell pepper, diced
1 jalapeño pepper, minced
3 cloves garlic, minced
1 (15-ounce) can no-salt-added black beans
½ cup corn kernels
2 tablespoons no-salt-added tomato paste
2 tablespoons Salt-Free Chili Seasoning (see Chapter 5)
½ cup nonfat sour cream
¼ cup chopped fresh cilantro

Salt-Free Chili Seasoning

Not all salt-free seasoning blends are the same, and nowhere is this more apparent than when it comes to chili seasonings. Some brands are fiery, while others are fairly bland. Taste seasonings before adding them to food. Carefully assess how much or how little needs to be added to your food and you'll never risk overseasoning.

1. Warm corn tortillas as desired; set aside.

2. Wash the chicken and cut into bite-sized pieces.

3. Heat a sauté pan over medium heat. Add the broth, carrot, and sweet potato, cover the pan, and cook for 5 minutes.

4. Add the chicken, onion, peppers, and garlic, cover, and cook for another 5 minutes, stirring once halfway through cooking time.

5. Add the beans with liquid, corn, tomato paste, and chili seasoning to the pan. Stir well and cook, stirring, for 5 minutes.

6. Remove from heat. Spoon filling into warm tortillas and garnish with sour cream and cilantro.

7. Serve immediately.

PER SERVING | Calories: 338 | Fat: 3 g | Protein: 17 g | Sodium: 90 mg | Fiber: 9 g | Carbohydrates: 63 g | Sugar: 5 g

Saucy Barbecued Chicken with Rice

A simple and satisfying low-sodium chicken recipe, full of BBQ deliciousness and amazingly tender meat. Serve as suggested or spoon over baked potatoes.

INGREDIENTS | SERVES 4

1 pound boneless, skinless chicken thighs

1 teaspoon canola oil

1 small onion, finely diced

2 cloves garlic, minced

1 large bell pepper, diced

2 (8-ounce) cans no-salt-added tomato sauce

2 tablespoons apple cider vinegar

2 tablespoons molasses

1 tablespoon honey

1 teaspoon liquid smoke

1½ teaspoons ground cumin

1 teaspoon ground sweet paprika

½ teaspoon dried oregano

½ teaspoon freshly ground black pepper

¼ teaspoon ground cayenne pepper

¼ cup chopped fresh cilantro

4 cups cooked brown rice

1. Wash chicken and pat dry. Cut thighs into bite-sized pieces and set aside.

2. Heat oil in a sauté pan over medium heat. Add the onion and garlic and sauté for 2 minutes.

3. Add the chicken and bell pepper and sauté for 2 minutes more.

4. Stir in the tomato sauce, vinegar, molasses, honey, liquid smoke, cumin, paprika, oregano, black pepper, and cayenne and stir to combine. Bring to a boil. Once boiling, lower heat to medium-low, cover, and simmer until chicken is cooked through, about 10–15 minutes.

5. Remove from heat. Stir in cilantro. Serve immediately, spooned over cooked rice.

PER SERVING | Calories: 474 | Fat: 7 g | Protein: 29 g | Sodium: 126 mg | Fiber: 6 g | Carbohydrates: 70 g | Sugar: 18 g

Spicy Yogurt–Marinated Chicken Tenders

Though this recipe uses chicken tenders, the marinade works equally well with any cut of chicken, from bone-in breasts to a whole roaster. For maximum impact, allow the chicken to steep as long as possible, even overnight. Recipe adapted from Stonyfield.com.

INGREDIENTS | SERVES 4

¾ cup nonfat plain yogurt

1 medium onion, finely chopped

3 cloves garlic, finely chopped

Juice of 1 fresh lime

1 tablespoon honey

1 teaspoon ground sweet paprika

1 teaspoon ground cumin

¼ teaspoon ground cayenne

¼ teaspoon ground cinnamon

1 pound boneless chicken tenders

Different Types of Marinades

Marinades can be divided into one of three types. Acidic marinades are those made with fruit juice, wine, or vinegar. Enzymatic marinades rely on fruit enzymes, such as those found in papaya, pineapple, or kiwi. Dairy-based marinades use either buttermilk or yogurt as their base. Of all three types, only dairy marinades reliably tenderize without the risk of toughening or disintegrating meat.

1. Measure all of the ingredients except the chicken into a mixing bowl and stir well to combine. Add the chicken and toss well to coat. Cover and refrigerate 30 minutes to 12 hours.

2. Once ready to cook, preheat oven to 375°F. Line a baking sheet with parchment or aluminum foil and arrange chicken in a single layer.

3. Place baking sheet on middle rack in oven and bake until golden brown, 10–15 minutes.

4. Remove from oven and serve immediately.

PER SERVING | Calories: 181 | Fat: 2 g | Protein: 28 g | Sodium: 110 mg | Fiber: 0 g | Carbohydrates: 11 g | Sugar: 9 g

Oven-Baked Chicken Tenders

Low-sodium restaurant-style chicken tenders. Baked rather than fried, these crispy tenders are much lower in fat, but have a whole lot of flavor. These freeze wonderfully; place leftovers into an airtight container for later meals. Serve with salt-free ketchup, barbecue sauce, and honey for dipping.

INGREDIENTS | SERVES 8

3 pounds boneless, skinless chicken breast tenderloins
½ cup unbleached all-purpose flour
½ cup white whole-wheat flour
½ cup salt-free bread crumbs
2 teaspoons garlic powder
2 teaspoons onion powder
1 teaspoon ground sweet paprika
1 teaspoon freshly ground black pepper
½ cup low-fat milk
1 egg white

1. Preheat oven to 375°F. Take out a large baking sheet, cover with aluminum foil, spray lightly with oil, and set aside.

2. Wash the chicken and pat dry.

3. Combine the flours, bread crumbs, and seasonings in a large zip-top plastic bag. Seal and shake well to combine.

4. Whisk together the milk and egg white in a shallow bowl.

5. One piece at a time, dip the chicken into the milk mixture, then place in the flour bag, seal, and shake vigorously to coat. Place breaded tenders on the prepared baking sheet.

6. Place baking sheet on middle rack in oven and bake for 10–15 minutes, until golden brown.

7. Remove from oven and serve immediately.

PER SERVING | Calories: 266 | Fat: 2 g | Protein: 45 g | Sodium: 132 mg | Fiber: 1 g | Carbohydrates: 13 g | Sugar: 1 g

Chicken with Rice, Lemon, and Kale

An oven-baked meal of hearty kale, meaty chunks of chicken, and rice bathed in a lemony broth.

INGREDIENTS | SERVES 4

8 boneless, skinless chicken thighs

1 cup basmati rice, rinsed

4 cups chopped fresh kale

2 shallots, chopped

2 cups low-sodium chicken broth

½ cup white wine

Juice and grated zest of 1 fresh lemon

4 cloves garlic, minced

1 tablespoon fresh thyme or 1 teaspoon dried

Freshly ground black pepper, to taste

Cooking with Wine

Wine can add depth and interest to many foods, and this is especially true when it comes to salt-free cooking. If you're wary of wine's intoxicating effects, add only to foods that will be heated. The cooking process evaporates the alcohol, leaving only its flavor behind. Fine wines are to be savored, and are best consumed by the glass. When cooking with wine, opt for inexpensive bottles.

1. Preheat oven to 425°F. Spray a 9" × 13" casserole pan lightly with oil.

2. Rinse the chicken and cut into bite-sized pieces. Arrange in a single layer in the prepared pan. Scatter the rice, kale, and shallots over top.

3. Add the broth, wine, lemon juice and zest, minced garlic, and thyme into a mixing bowl and whisk well to combine. Carefully pour the mixture over the contents of the pan. Season with freshly ground black pepper, to taste.

4. Cover pan tightly with aluminum foil, then place on middle rack in oven and bake for 30 minutes. Remove from oven and serve immediately.

PER SERVING | Calories: 340 | Fat: 5 g | Protein: 24 g | Sodium: 140 mg | Fiber: 2 g | Carbohydrates: 45 g | Sugar: <1 g

Honey Mustard Chicken Breasts

Hey mustard lovers! This moist and flavorful recipe will leave you wanting more. Although boneless breasts are used here for ease, substitute whatever chicken parts you have on hand; just remember to adjust the cooking time accordingly.

INGREDIENTS | SERVES 4

1 pound boneless, skinless chicken breasts
2 tablespoons mustard seeds
1 tablespoon ground dry mustard
1 tablespoon distilled white vinegar
2 tablespoons water
¼ cup white wine
2 tablespoons honey

1. Wash the chicken breasts and pat dry.

2. Crush the mustard seeds slightly using a mortar and pestle or small spice grinder.

3. Place the seeds and remaining ingredients into a bowl or plastic zip-top bag and mix well to combine.

4. Add the chicken to the marinade and coat completely. Cover bowl or seal bag tightly and refrigerate several hours or overnight.

5. If grilling, preheat grill. Remove breasts from the marinade, place on grill, and cook, turning once, until chicken is slightly crisp outside and no longer pink inside, about 10–15 minutes per side.

6. To bake the chicken, preheat oven to 375°F. Place the breasts in a baking pan, along with a little of the marinade. Cover pan tightly with foil. Place pan on middle rack in oven and bake until chicken reaches an internal temperature of 160°F, about 30 minutes.

7. Remove from oven or grill and serve immediately.

PER SERVING | Calories: 170 | Fat: 1 g | Protein: 26 g | Sodium: 103 mg | Fiber: 0 g | Carbohydrates: 9 g | Sugar: 8 g

Chicken Curry with Creamy Tomato Sauce

This quick and easy chicken curry tastes terrific and will leave your house smelling glorious. Serve over cooked basmati rice.

INGREDIENTS | SERVES 4

1 pound boneless, skinless chicken breasts

1 teaspoon canola oil

1 large onion, diced

3 cloves garlic, minced

1 tablespoon minced fresh ginger

1 jalapeño pepper, minced

1 (15-ounce) can no-salt-added diced tomatoes

2 tablespoons tomato paste

¾ cup low-sodium chicken or vegetable broth

½ cup nonfat plain yogurt

2 teaspoons salt-free garam masala or curry powder

½ teaspoon ground sweet paprika

¼ teaspoon freshly ground black pepper

¼ cup chopped fresh cilantro

1. Wash chicken breasts and pat dry. Cut into bite-sized chunks and set aside.

2. Heat oil in a large sauté pan over medium heat. Add chicken, onion, garlic, and ginger and cook, stirring, for 5 minutes.

3. Add the jalapeño, tomatoes with juice, tomato paste, broth, yogurt, garam masala, paprika, and pepper and stir to combine. Bring to a boil.

4. Once boiling, reduce heat to medium-low, cover, and simmer, stirring frequently, until chicken is fully cooked, about 20 minutes.

5. Remove from heat. Stir in the cilantro and serve immediately.

PER SERVING | Calories: 189 | Fat: 3 g | Protein: 29 g | Sodium: 130 mg | Fiber: 1 g | Carbohydrates: 10 g | Sugar: 6 g

Chicken Facts

Chicken's mild flavor and affordable nature make it one of the most popular types of protein worldwide. When preparing chicken, first remove the skin; this will greatly reduce the amount of fat you're consuming. White meat contains less fat than dark meat, but dark meat contains a higher concentration of some nutrients. Skinless chicken is an excellent source of protein, vitamin B_6, and minerals.

Low-Sodium Kung Pao Chicken

The spicy bite of ginger, the tang of rice wine vinegar, the smoky depth of sesame oil, that certain indescribable something that says "I am Chinese takeout," it's all here! Adapted from Fine Cooking.

INGREDIENTS | SERVES 4

1 cup low-sodium chicken broth

2 tablespoons Faux Soy Sauce (see Chapter 5)

1 tablespoon balsamic vinegar

5 tablespoons cornstarch, divided

2 teaspoons sesame oil

1 teaspoon sugar

1 pound boneless, skinless chicken breasts, cubed

¼ teaspoon freshly ground black pepper

2 tablespoons canola oil, divided

¼ teaspoon dried red pepper flakes

2 tablespoons minced fresh ginger

6 scallions, sliced, whites and greens kept separate

1 medium red bell pepper, cubed

2 medium stalks celery, sliced

2 medium carrots, sliced

¼ cup plain unflavored rice vinegar

¼ cup unsalted cashews or peanuts, chopped

1. Place the chicken broth, Faux Soy Sauce, balsamic vinegar, 1 tablespoon cornstarch, sesame oil, and sugar into a bowl. Whisk well to combine and set aside.

2. Place the chicken into a mixing bowl, add 4 tablespoons cornstarch and black pepper, to taste, and toss well to coat using a pair of tongs.

3. Heat 1 tablespoon oil in a sauté pan over medium heat. Add the chicken and cook until lightly browned on all sides, about 4 minutes total.

4. Add the remaining tablespoon oil to the pan. Add the red pepper flakes, ginger, and whites of the scallions and cook, stirring, for 1 minute.

5. Add the bell pepper, celery, and carrots and sauté until they soften slightly, about 2 minutes.

6. Add the rice vinegar and scrape the bottom of the pan to incorporate any browned bits.

7. Give the chicken broth mixture a quick whisk, then add to the pan.

8. Check the chicken. If still pink inside, reduce heat and cook a couple minutes more. Remove pan from heat and serve immediately, sprinkled with the chopped nuts and scallion greens.

PER SERVING | Calories: 347 | Fat: 14 g | Protein: 29 g | Sodium: 135 mg | Fiber: 2 g | Carbohydrates: 24 g | Sugar: 8 g

CHAPTER 13

Vegan and Vegetarian Dishes

30-Minute Vegetarian Pizza

*In one word: YUM! Make it vegan by using ¼ cup nutritional yeast flakes,
egg replacement powder, and nondairy milk instead of the animal products.
An equally good gluten-free version can be made using brown rice flour.
The GF crust has a tendency to stick, however, so make sure the pan is well oiled and floured.*

INGREDIENTS | SERVES 4

1 cup white whole-wheat flour

1 teaspoon all-purpose salt-free seasoning

1 teaspoon salt-free Italian seasoning

½ teaspoon garlic powder

2 egg whites

⅔ cup low-fat milk

2 teaspoons olive oil

1 small eggplant, peeled and diced

1 medium onion, diced

½ cup no-salt-added pasta sauce

1 small bell pepper, diced

1 small tomato, diced

1 cup sliced mushrooms

½ cup chopped fresh broccoli

2 cloves garlic, minced

2 tablespoons chopped fresh basil

½ cup shredded Swiss cheese

1. Preheat oven to 425°F. Grease and flour a 12-inch nonstick pizza pan and set aside.

2. Place the flour and seasonings into a mixing bowl and whisk well to combine. Add the egg whites and milk and stir well. Pour batter into the prepared pizza pan and set aside.

3. Place a large skillet over medium heat. Add the diced eggplant and onion and cook, stirring, for 5 minutes.

4. Remove from heat and spoon mixture evenly over the batter in the pan. Place pan on middle rack in oven and bake for 20 minutes.

5. Once crust is baked spread pasta sauce evenly over crust. Top pizza with bell pepper, tomato, mushrooms, broccoli, garlic, and basil. Sprinkle the Swiss cheese evenly over top.

6. Return pan to oven and bake 3–5 minutes, until cheese has melted.

7. Remove pizza from oven. Gently remove from pan and cut into 8 slices. Serve immediately.

PER SERVING | Calories: 242 | Fat: 7 g | Protein: 13 g | Sodium: 82 mg | Fiber: 6 g | Carbohydrates: 34 g | Sugar: 7 g

Mac and Peas and Carrots

Satisfy cravings with this vegan spin on comfort food. Whole-grain macaroni, tender peas, and carrots tossed with a creamy, heart-healthy, dairy-free sauce.

INGREDIENTS | SERVES 6

1 pound whole-grain macaroni

¼ cup walnuts

2 cloves garlic

1 teaspoon salt-free prepared mustard

1 teaspoon freshly squeezed lemon juice

¼ cup nutritional yeast flakes

¾ cup low-sodium vegetable broth, divided

1 medium onion, diced

3 medium carrots, diced

1½ cups frozen peas

It's All about Perspective

Healthy dieting is about sacrifice and reward. In return for giving up certain foods, your body is able to heal and return to a rejuvenated state of being. Saying goodbye to favorite foods can be hard, but when you focus on all that you receive in return, it's not so difficult. When cravings for forbidden foods arise, remind yourself why you are no longer consuming them, and reward yourself with something else, like a walk in the park, a trip to the library, or a new music CD. You can find enjoyment in many ways other than food, and live a longer, happier life in the process.

1. Cook macaroni according to package directions, omitting salt. Drain and set aside.

2. Measure the walnuts, garlic, mustard, lemon juice, and nutritional yeast into a food processor and pulse to combine. Add ¼ cup of the broth and purée. Set aside.

3. Heat the remaining broth in a sauté pan over medium heat. Add the onion and carrots and cook, stirring, for 7 minutes.

4. Add the peas and continue to cook, stirring, for 3 minutes.

5. Remove pan from heat. Add pasta and sauce and stir well to combine. Serve immediately.

PER SERVING | Calories: 319 | Fat: 4 g | Protein: 15 g | Sodium: 48 mg | Fiber: 9 g | Carbohydrates: 58 g | Sugar: 5 g

Sesame Tofu with Sautéed Green Beans

A fantastic vegetarian dish for those wanting something meaty. The baked tofu is toothsome and dense, and the sautéed green beans have an irresistible crunch. It's a meal you can sink your teeth into, literally!

INGREDIENTS | SERVES 4

1 pound extra-firm tofu
1 tablespoon sesame oil
2 tablespoons toasted sesame seeds
Freshly ground black pepper, to taste
1 pound fresh green beans
1 teaspoon sesame oil
1 medium red onion, diced
3 cloves garlic, minced
1 tablespoon minced fresh ginger

1. Preheat oven to 425°F. Spray a baking sheet lightly with oil and set aside.

2. Drain the tofu and press gently between paper towels to release excess water.

3. Cut the tofu crosswise into 6 equal sections, then turn each section over to lay flat. Slice each section in half lengthwise, leaving 12 (1" × 3½") pieces.

4. Cut each piece in half crosswise; you will now have 24 (1" × 1¾") pieces.

5. Place tofu in a bowl, add oil, and toss gently to coat using your (freshly washed) hands. Arrange tofu on the prepared baking sheet and sprinkle evenly with sesame seeds and freshly ground pepper, to taste.

6. Place baking sheet on middle rack in oven and bake for 25–30 minutes, turning the tofu once halfway through cooking time.

7. While tofu is baking, wash and trim beans, then cut into roughly 2-inch pieces.

8. Heat 1 teaspoon of sesame oil in a sauté pan over medium heat. Add the onion, garlic, and ginger and sauté for 2 minutes.

9. Add the beans and sauté for 5–8 minutes.

10. Remove tofu from the oven and add to the pan. Stir to coat, season to taste with freshly ground black pepper, and serve immediately.

PER SERVING | Calories: 238 | Fat: 12 g | Protein: 15 g | Sodium: 20 mg | Fiber: 6 g | Carbohydrates: 19 g | Sugar: 6 g

Whole-Grain Penne with Lemony Roasted Asparagus

Such fabulous flavor with so few ingredients! Oven roasting draws out depth in the vegetables, punctuated by the citrus burst. If you don't have penne, substitute another favorite pasta.

INGREDIENTS | SERVES 6

1½ pounds fresh asparagus
8 ounces mushrooms, thickly sliced
1 medium red onion, diced
1 tablespoon olive oil
Juice and grated zest of 1 fresh lemon
¼ teaspoon freshly ground black pepper
1 package dry whole-grain penne
2 tablespoons chopped fresh dill

Roasting for Flavor

Roasting is simply cooking food at a very high temperature. You can roast in an oven, or you can roast over an open flame. Oven roasting allows for convenience and control. You're able to adjust not only the temperature of the oven but the proximity of the food to the flame. The roasting process allows the natural sugars present in many foods to caramelize, leaving the cooked versions much sweeter and more complex than they were when raw.

1. Preheat oven to 450°F. Line a large baking sheet with aluminum foil and set aside.

2. Trim woody ends from asparagus and cut stalks into 2-inch pieces. Place in a mixing bowl with mushrooms and onion. Add oil, 2 tablespoons lemon juice, and black pepper and toss to coat.

3. Spread onto the prepared baking sheet. Place on middle rack in oven and bake for 20 minutes.

4. Cook penne according to package directions, omitting salt. Drain.

5. Once vegetables are roasted, add to pasta, along with all the cooking juices. Add remaining lemon juice and zest and toss to coat. Season with additional black pepper, to taste, and fresh dill. Serve immediately.

PER SERVING | Calories: 305 | Fat: 3 g | Protein: 14 g | Sodium: 27 mg | Fiber: 12 g | Carbohydrates: 60 g | Sugar: 6 g

Tofu Stroganoff

If you like the combination of creamy sauce, mushrooms, and noodles found in classic Beef Stroganoff, you'll love this updated salt-free version made with tofu. Adapted from Vegetarian Times.

INGREDIENTS | SERVES 6

1 pound wide yolkless egg noodles
1 pound extra-firm tofu
4 teaspoons olive oil, divided
1 large onion, diced
4 cloves garlic, minced
3 cups sliced baby bella mushrooms
¼ cup sliced fresh chives
½ teaspoon freshly ground black pepper
¾ cup nonfat sour cream
3 tablespoons low-sodium soy sauce

1. Cook noodles according to package directions, omitting salt. Drain and set aside.

2. Drain tofu and gently press between paper towels to release as much liquid as possible.

3. Slice tofu into long strips, about 3" × ¾" × ½" in height. Set aside.

4. Heat 2 teaspoons olive oil in a sauté pan over medium heat. Add onion, garlic, and mushrooms and cook, stirring, for 8 minutes.

5. Add chives and pepper and stir. Remove mixture from pan and set aside.

6. Return pan to medium heat and add remaining oil. Add tofu and cook until golden brown, about 8 minutes.

7. Return the mushroom mixture to the pan, add sour cream and soy sauce, and stir gently. Cook 2 minutes.

8. Remove from heat and spoon over egg noodles. Serve immediately.

PER SERVING | Calories: 432 | Fat: 12 g | Protein: 20 g | Sodium: 62 mg | Fiber: 5 g | Carbohydrates: 59 g | Sugar: 4 g

Pesto Rice with Portabella Mushrooms

A one-pot vegetarian meal, perfect for potluck parties. Best made with white basmati rice, but equally delicious with your choice of whole-grain pasta.

INGREDIENTS | SERVES 6

2 cups basmati rice

3 cups water

1 tablespoon olive oil

1 medium onion, chopped

2 cloves garlic, minced

8 ounces baby bella mushrooms

6 tablespoons Basil Pesto
(see Chapter 5)

Freshly ground black pepper, to taste

Rice Tip

If you have the time, soak your basmati rice for 30 minutes before cooking. Measure rice into a fine-mesh sieve and rinse repeatedly under cool running water. Place rice into cooking pot, add desired amount of water, and let sit. The soaking water can be used to cook the rice, with no draining necessary. This soaking process will enhance the flavor and texture of the rice.

1. Measure rice into a fine-mesh sieve and rinse well under cold running water. If time permits, let the rice sit for 30 minutes before cooking. If not, transfer rice to a saucepan and add water. Place pot over medium-high heat and bring to a boil. As soon as water begins to boil, immediately reduce heat to low, cover, and simmer for 15 minutes.

2. Once rice is cooked, remove pot from heat and fluff rice using a fork. Set aside.

3. Heat the oil in a sauté pan over medium heat. Add the onion and garlic and cook, stirring, for 2 minutes.

4. Add the mushrooms and sauté until tender, about 4 minutes. Remove from heat.

5. Add rice to the pan, along with the prepared pesto. Stir well to combine. Season with freshly ground black pepper, to taste. Serve immediately.

PER SERVING | Calories: 291 | Fat: 9 g | Protein: 6 g | Sodium: 21 mg | Fiber: 2 g | Carbohydrates: 44 g | Sugar: 1 g

Spicy Chickpea Tacos with Arugula

These may be vegan, but they're the tastiest tacos ever! A thick and spicy sauce dotted with meaty garbanzos, the peppery cool of arugula, and crunchy bite of corn. Spoon extra filling over cooked brown rice if you run short of packaged shells.

INGREDIENTS | SERVES 6

1 package low-sodium taco shells
6 cups fresh baby arugula
3 cups cooked no-salt-added garbanzo beans
4 tablespoons salt-free tomato paste
1 (8-ounce) can no-salt-added tomato sauce
1 tablespoon apple cider vinegar
1 tablespoon light brown sugar
2 teaspoons salt-free chili seasoning
1 teaspoon ground dry mustard
1 teaspoon onion powder
½ teaspoon garlic powder
¼–½ teaspoon freshly ground black pepper
⅛–¼ teaspoon dried red pepper flakes

1. Heat taco shells according to package directions.

2. Wash the arugula and pat dry. Set aside.

3. In a saucepan, measure remaining ingredients and stir well to combine.

4. Place pan over medium heat and simmer, stirring frequently, for 10 minutes. Remove from heat.

5. Fill warm taco shells with arugula and spoon bean mixture over top. Serve immediately.

PER SERVING | Calories: 288 | Fat: 8 g | Protein: 10 g | Sodium: 30 mg | Fiber: 9 g | Carbohydrates: 46 g | Sugar: 10 g

Vegetable Fried Rice

Thanks to low-sodium soy sauce, garlic, and ginger, this vegetarian fried rice has authentic taste without the health hazard. Add tofu and/or chopped nuts for added heft and protein if desired.

INGREDIENTS | SERVES 4

1 tablespoon sesame oil
1 medium onion, diced
3 medium carrots, sliced
1 bunch fresh broccoli, cut into florets
2 cups sugar snap peas or snow pea pods
3 cloves garlic, minced
1 tablespoon minced fresh ginger
4 cups cooked brown rice
1 tablespoon low-sodium soy sauce
½ teaspoon freshly ground black pepper

1. Heat oil in a wok over medium. When oil begins to sizzle, add vegetables, garlic, and ginger and cook, stirring, for 5 minutes.

2. Add rice, soy sauce, and black pepper and cook, stirring, another 5 minutes.

3. Remove from heat and serve immediately.

PER SERVING | Calories: 341 | Fat: 6 g | Protein: 10 g | Sodium: 94 mg | Fiber: 9 g | Carbohydrates: 64 g | Sugar: 8 g

Kale Stuffed Manicotti

A vegan version of the classic Italian dish. Spinach, Swiss chard, or another dark leafy green may be substituted for the kale.

INGREDIENTS | SERVES 6

1 package dried manicotti
1 medium onion, chopped
3 cloves garlic, minced
7 cups chopped fresh kale
1 pound firm tofu, drained
1 teaspoon dried Italian seasoning
¼ teaspoon freshly ground black pepper
⅛ teaspoon dried red pepper flakes
3 cups no-salt-added pasta sauce
2 tablespoons nutritional yeast flakes (e.g., Red Star)

Nutritional Yeast Flakes

Nutritional yeast is a type of inactive yeast with a zingy, cheese-like flavor, making it a great stand-in for Parmesan cheese in low-sodium and vegan diets. The little yellow flakes can be sprinkled on popcorn, pasta, anything you'd like to perk up. Nutritional yeast contains important vitamins, such as vitamin B_{12}, often found in meat, so is an especially nutritious supplement for vegetarians and vegans. Nutritional yeast is sold at Whole Foods markets, many natural food stores, and online. Red Star is an excellent brand, as is Bragg.

1. Preheat oven to 400°F. Get out a 9" × 13" baking pan and set aside.

2. Cook manicotti according to package directions, omitting salt. Drain and set aside.

3. While pasta is cooking, assemble filling. In a stockpot over medium heat, place onion and garlic and sauté until soft, about 3 minutes.

4. Add kale and cook, stirring, for 4–5 minutes more. Remove pot from heat and transfer contents to a food processor.

5. Pulse until smooth. Add tofu and seasonings and pulse until smooth.

6. Spread a thin layer of sauce into the bottom of the baking pan. Fill manicotti and arrange in the pan. Pour remaining pasta sauce over the manicotti and sprinkle with the nutritional yeast.

7. Cover pan with aluminum foil, place on middle rack in oven, and bake until hot and bubbly, about 20–30 minutes.

8. Remove from oven and serve immediately.

PER SERVING | Calories: 441 | Fat: 6 g | Protein: 2 g | Sodium: 51 mg | Fiber: 7 g | Carbohydrates: 77 g | Sugar: 8 g

Quinoa with Mixed Veggies and Cilantro Peanut Pesto

Creamy and filling, like a quinoa risotto, this hearty one-dish meal has a fabulous combination of flavors. Because it's vegan, and uses quinoa (a gluten-free grain), it's a great choice for parties and other group events.

INGREDIENTS | SERVES 6

1 cup quinoa

2 cups water

1 teaspoon olive oil

1 medium red onion, diced

2 medium carrots, diced

8 ounces mushrooms, chopped

1 medium red bell pepper, diced

3 tablespoons Cilantro Peanut Pesto (see Chapter 5)

2 scallions, sliced

Freshly ground black pepper, to taste

An Important Note about Quinoa

Quinoa has a bitter-tasting outer coating on its grains that must be removed prior to cooking. Many brands of commercial quinoa remove this prior to packaging, so you can simply measure the quinoa and cook. But if you're not using organic, prewashed quinoa, don't forget to rinse well prior to cooking.

1. Measure the quinoa into a saucepan. Add water and bring to a boil over high heat. Once boiling, reduce heat to medium-low, cover, and simmer for 15 minutes.

2. Heat oil in a sauté pan over medium heat. Add the onion and sauté for 2 minutes.

3. Add carrots, mushrooms, and bell pepper and cook, stirring, for 8 minutes. Remove from heat.

4. Stir in the cooked quinoa and pesto. Sprinkle with the scallions and season with freshly ground black pepper, to taste. Serve immediately.

PER SERVING | Calories: 204 | Fat: 4 g | Protein: 7 g | Sodium: 59 mg | Fiber: 5 g | Carbohydrates: 35 g | Sugar: 5 g

Quick and Healthy Eggplant Parmesan

From its crisp eggplant croutons and fresh basil taste to its 15-minute preparation time, this guilt-free version of the perennial favorite will please picky eaters and cooks alike. Nutritional yeast may be substituted for the grated cheese.

INGREDIENTS | SERVES 4

1 package dry whole-grain pasta
1 medium eggplant
¼ cup salt-free bread crumbs
1 teaspoon dried Italian seasoning
¼ teaspoon freshly ground black pepper
1 tablespoon olive oil
2 cups no-salt-added pasta sauce
2 tablespoons grated Parmesan cheese
2 tablespoons chopped fresh basil

1. Cook pasta according to package directions, omitting salt. While pasta is cooking, prepare the eggplant.

2. Preheat oven to 425°F. Spray a sided baking sheet lightly with oil and set aside.

3. Peel eggplant and cut into 1-inch cubes. Place into a large mixing bowl. Add bread crumbs, seasoning, pepper, and oil. Toss well to coat.

4. Arrange in a single layer on prepared baking sheet. Place on middle rack in oven and bake for 10 minutes.

5. Remove pan from oven. Top pasta with the baked eggplant and cover with sauce, cheese, and basil. Serve immediately.

PER SERVING | Calories: 480 | Fat: 6 g | Protein: 18 g | Sodium: 62 mg | Fiber: 15 g | Carbohydrates: 94 g | Sugar: 10 g

10-Minute Thai Noodles

These spicy noodles will satisfy your hunger for something healthy and filling like nothing else. Unsalted chunky peanut butter is specified; feel free to substitute creamy peanut butter and a tablespoon of chopped unsalted peanuts if you prefer.

INGREDIENTS | SERVES 6

1 pound dry angel hair or capellini pasta

3 teaspoons sesame oil, divided

1 small red onion, diced

4 garlic cloves, minced

1 tablespoon minced fresh ginger

1 medium red bell pepper, diced

½ cup low-sodium vegetable broth

2 tablespoons unsalted chunky peanut butter

2 tablespoons freshly squeezed lime juice

½ teaspoon dried red pepper flakes

3 scallions, sliced

1. Cook pasta according to package directions, omitting salt. Drain. Add 1 teaspoon sesame oil to cooked pasta and toss well to coat. Set aside.

2. Heat remaining 2 teaspoons oil in a sauté pan over medium heat. Add onion, garlic, and ginger and sauté for 2 minutes.

3. Add bell pepper and sauté for 3 minutes. Remove from heat.

4. Stir in broth, peanut butter, lime juice, red pepper flakes, and scallions.

5. Add pasta and toss well to coat. Serve immediately.

PER SERVING | Calories: 377 | Fat: 6 g | Protein: 13 g | Sodium: 20 mg | Fiber: 5 g | Carbohydrates: 66 g | Sugar: 5 g

Unsalted Peanut Butter

Many supermarkets as well as natural food stores, Whole Foods, and Trader Joe's sell unsalted peanut butter. Some stores are even installing their own grinding machines, so you can get the freshest, salt-free peanut butter imaginable. If you cannot locate any locally, unsalted peanut butter is sold online. The vast majority of peanuts in the United States are grown using chemical pesticides; purchase organic, unsalted peanut butter whenever possible.

Asparagus, Swiss, and Ricotta Frittata

Frittatas are impressive, yet ridiculously easy to make. Liquid egg replacement is stocked beside the eggs in most supermarkets.

INGREDIENTS | SERVES 4

8 stalks fresh asparagus

1 shallot, finely diced

1¼ cups liquid egg replacement (e.g., Egg Beaters)

¼ cup Roasted Red Peppers (see Chapter 15), sliced

¼ cup shredded Swiss cheese

1 tablespoon nonfat ricotta cheese

Freshly ground black pepper, to taste

1. Move rack to top of the oven and preheat to 450°F.

2. Trim the asparagus and cut into thirds. Steam the asparagus over high heat for 5 minutes.

3. Spray an ovenproof skillet with cooking oil. Place over medium heat, add shallot, and sauté for 2 minutes.

4. Add liquid egg replacement to pan and remove from heat.

5. Top with asparagus, red pepper, and Swiss. Dollop ricotta over top and season with freshly ground black pepper, to taste.

6. Place skillet on top rack in oven and bake for 10 minutes.

7. Remove from oven. Slide a heatproof spatula around and under frittata to loosen. Remove and cut into wedges. Serve immediately.

PER SERVING | Calories: 112 | Fat: 4 g | Protein: 13 g | Sodium: 161 mg | Fiber: 1 g | Carbohydrates: 4 g | Sugar: 2 g

Mushroom and Eggplant Curry

A salt-free curry that's brimming over with taste. The mushrooms and eggplant are so "meaty," you'll forget it's strictly vegan!

INGREDIENTS | SERVES 4

1 medium eggplant
1 teaspoon olive oil
1 medium red onion, diced
1 tablespoon minced fresh ginger
3 cloves garlic, minced
8 ounces white mushrooms, sliced
1 cup low-sodium vegetable broth
1 (15-ounce) can no-salt-added diced tomatoes
1 tablespoon salt-free curry powder
½ teaspoon freshly ground black pepper
¼ cup chopped fresh cilantro

Salt-Free Seasonings Alert

Salt is cheap and abundant, making it an inexpensive way for manufacturers to bulk up their herb and spice blends. It's important to be mindful of this when shopping for salt-free seasonings. Salt may not be advertised on the front of the package, but is often included in the list of ingredients on the back. Check labels carefully. Unless something is specifically labeled salt free, it very well may not be.

1. Peel eggplant and cut into 1-inch cubes.

2. Heat oil in a large skillet or sauté pan over medium heat. Add the onion, ginger, and garlic and sauté for 2 minutes.

3. Add eggplant and mushrooms and cook, stirring, for 3 minutes.

4. Add broth and cook for 1 minute, stirring and scraping to get all of the brown bits off the bottom of the pan.

5. Add tomatoes with juice and curry powder and stir well to combine. Reduce heat to low, cover, and simmer for 10 minutes, stirring once or twice.

6. Remove from heat. Stir in ground pepper and cilantro. Serve immediately.

PER SERVING | Calories: 67 | Fat: 2 g | Protein: 3 g | Sodium: 50 mg | Fiber: 3 g | Carbohydrates: 12 g | Sugar: 4 g

Super Yummy Meatless Meatloaf

A main course certain to please meat eaters and vegetarians alike, this meatless meatloaf is moist, melt-in-your-mouth comfort food. Substitute 3 cups cooked mashed potatoes and 1½ cups rolled or quick oats for the bulgur for a gluten-free meatloaf. Adapted from The Complete Cooking Light Cookbook.

INGREDIENTS | SERVES 6

1 cup dry bulgur wheat

3 cups boiling water

1 (15-ounce) can no-salt-added kidney beans

1 small red onion, diced

1 small–medium bell pepper, diced

1 small stalk celery

3 garlic cloves, minced

¼ cup chopped fresh cilantro

1½ teaspoons ground cumin

1 teaspoon salt-free chili seasoning

½ cup low-sodium barbecue sauce, divided

¼ cup salt-free ketchup

3 teaspoons salt-free mustard

Freshly ground black pepper, to taste

1. Preheat oven to 450°F. Spray an 8-inch square pan lightly with oil and set aside.

2. Measure the bulgur into a saucepan and stir in the boiling water. Bring to a boil over high heat, then reduce heat to low, cover, and simmer for 10 minutes. Drain any excess water. Set aside.

3. Drain the beans and rinse well. Mash using the tines of a fork and place into a large mixing bowl.

4. Add the cooked bulgur, onion, bell pepper, celery, garlic, cilantro, cumin, chili seasoning, ¼ cup barbecue sauce, ketchup, mustard, and black pepper, to taste. Mix together using your (freshly washed) hands, then transfer to the prepared pan and smooth to even.

5. Spoon the remaining ¼ cup barbecue sauce over top and spread evenly. Place pan on middle rack in oven and bake for 20 minutes.

6. Remove from oven. Cool briefly before slicing into portions and serving.

PER SERVING | Calories: 190 | Fat: 1 g | Protein: 9 g | Sodium: 15 mg | Fiber: 9 g | Carbohydrates: 38 g | Sugar: 4 g

Zucchini Cakes

These scrumptious oven-baked patties are a perfect way to use some of your garden surplus. Garnish with homemade horseradish sauce or salt-free ketchup. Substitute your favorite salt-free seasoning blend for the all-purpose seasoning if desired.

INGREDIENTS | SERVES 4

1 medium zucchini, shredded (with skin)

1 small red onion, finely diced

1 egg white

¾ cup salt-free bread crumbs

2 teaspoons salt-free all-purpose seasoning

Freshly ground black pepper, to taste

Homemade Horseradish Sauce

Combine 2 tablespoons store-bought horseradish with ¼ cup nonfat sour cream. Add 1–2 tablespoons of chopped fresh herbs, such as dill or chives, a minced clove of garlic, and freshly ground black pepper to taste. Use immediately or cover and refrigerate until ready to serve.

1. Preheat oven to 400°F. Spray a baking sheet lightly with oil and set aside.

2. Press shredded zucchini gently between paper towels to release excess liquid.

3. In a large bowl, combine zucchini, onion, egg, bread crumbs, seasoning, and black pepper, to taste. Mix well.

4. Shape mixture into patties and place on the prepared baking sheet.

5. Place baking sheet on middle rack in oven and bake for 10 minutes. Gently flip patties and return to oven to bake for another 10 minutes.

6. Remove from oven and serve immediately.

PER SERVING | Calories: 94 | Fat: 1 g | Protein: 4 g | Sodium: 22 mg | Fiber: 2 g | Carbohydrates: 19 g | Sugar: 2 g

Amazing Veggie Casserole with Tofu Topping

The recipe makes use of some of the healthiest and least expensive veggies: carrots, onions, cabbage, and kale. Add a topping of crumbled extra-firm tofu, bread crumbs, and chopped nuts and you've got an irresistible casserole even skeptics will love. Serve over cooked brown rice. Adapted from Gourmet Magazine.

INGREDIENTS | SERVES 8

2 teaspoons olive oil

2 medium onions, sliced thinly

½ medium head green cabbage, sliced

1 pound kale, leaves only, chopped

3 medium carrots, sliced into thin sticks

½ cup low-sodium vegetable broth or water

2 tablespoons low-sodium soy sauce

1½ cups salt-free bread crumbs

8 ounces extra-firm tofu

¼ cup chopped walnuts

2 garlic cloves

2 tablespoons olive oil

2 teaspoons dried basil

1½ teaspoons dried oregano

1 teaspoon ground sweet paprika

1. Preheat oven to 350°F. Get out a 9" × 13" baking pan and set aside.

2. Heat oil in a large sauté pan over medium heat. Add onion and cook, stirring, for 2 minutes.

3. Add cabbage, kale, carrots, broth, and soy sauce. Cover the pan and cook, stirring occasionally, for 10 minutes. Transfer contents to the baking pan and set aside.

4. To make the topping, measure remaining ingredients into a food processor and pulse to combine. Sprinkle over vegetables in baking dish.

5. Place dish on middle rack in oven and bake, uncovered, until topping is golden brown and vegetables are heated through, about 15–20 minutes.

6. Remove from oven and serve immediately.

PER SERVING | Calories: 238 | Fat: 9 g | Protein: 10 g | Sodium: 69 mg | Fiber: 6 g | Carbohydrates: 33 g | Sugar: 6 g

Crustless Spinach Pie

A deliciously light vegetarian entrée. Its quiche-like appeal is addictive, each bite filled with toothsome rice and spinach in a peppery custard, but without the added fat and chore of a crust.

INGREDIENTS | SERVES 8

2 teaspoons olive oil
1 medium red onion, diced
3 cloves garlic, minced
10 ounces fresh baby spinach
1½ cups cooked rice
½ cup low-fat milk
2 eggs, beaten well
1 tablespoon grated Parmesan cheese
½ teaspoon freshly ground black pepper

Eat Your Spinach!

Spinach is low in calories, high in fiber and protein, and an excellent source of vitamins A, B$_6$, C, E, and K. Spinach also contains many important minerals as well as disease-fighting antioxidants. It's easy to grow at home, can be eaten fresh or frozen, raw or cooked, in both savory dishes as well as sweets. Try it in a delicious Green Mango Smoothie (see Chapter 6).

1. Preheat oven to 350°F. Spray a pie pan lightly with oil and set aside.

2. Heat oil in a sauté pan over medium heat. Add onion and garlic and sauté for 2 minutes.

3. Add the spinach and continue to cook, stirring, until spinach has wilted fully, about 3–5 minutes.

4. Remove from heat and transfer to a mixing bowl. Add the cooked rice to the bowl and stir. Add the remaining ingredients and stir well to combine.

5. Pour the mixture into the prepared pan and smooth to even. Place on middle rack in oven and bake for 25 minutes.

6. Remove from oven and cool 5 minutes before cutting and serving. Serve warm or at room temperature.

PER SERVING | Calories: 83 | Fat: 3 g | Protein: 4 g | Sodium: 63 mg | Fiber: 1 g | Carbohydrates: 10 g | Sugar: 1 g

Veggie Baked Ziti

Delicious comfort food at its low-sodium best, this version of baked ziti is packed with fresh veggies. Water-packed mozzarella is often sold in the specialty cheese section of supermarkets. It's softer and much lower in sodium than its dry counterparts. If you can't find it, substitute shredded Swiss cheese instead.

INGREDIENTS | SERVES 6

1 pound dry whole-grain ziti

1 tablespoon olive oil

1 medium onion, diced

4 cloves garlic, minced

1 medium bell pepper, diced

1 medium yellow squash, diced

1 medium zucchini, diced

1 (15-ounce) can no-salt-added diced tomatoes

2 (8-ounce) cans no-salt-added tomato sauce

2 tablespoons tomato paste

1 teaspoon brown sugar

1 teaspoon dried basil

½ teaspoon dried marjoram

½ teaspoon dried oregano

½ teaspoon freshly ground black pepper

¼ teaspoon dried savory

¼ teaspoon dried thyme

4 ounces fresh water-packed mozzarella cheese, shredded

2 tablespoons grated Parmesan cheese

1. Preheat oven to 400°F. Get out a 9" × 13" baking pan and set aside.

2. Cook ziti according to package directions, omitting salt. Drain and set aside.

3. Heat oil in a sauté pan over medium heat. Add onion and garlic and sauté for 2 minutes.

4. Add bell pepper, squash, zucchini, tomatoes with juice, tomato sauce, tomato paste, brown sugar, and seasonings and cook, stirring, for 10 minutes. Remove from heat.

5. Pour sauce into the pot of pasta. Add the cheeses and stir to combine. Pour mixture into the baking dish. Cover tightly with aluminum foil. Place pan on middle rack in oven and bake for 20 minutes.

6. Remove from oven and serve immediately.

PER SERVING | Calories: 384 | Fat: 8 g | Protein: 17 g | Sodium: 180 mg | Fiber: 11 g | Carbohydrates: 65 g | Sugar: 10 g

Linguine with Plum Tomatoes, Mushrooms, and Tempeh

Pasta is always an easy and filling dinner, especially for vegetarians, and this sauce adds a new dimension to standard low-sodium fare. The slight acidity of the tomatoes provides a wonderful contrast to the nutty, earthy flavors of the mushrooms and tempeh.

INGREDIENTS | SERVES 6

1 pound dry whole-grain linguine

1 (28-ounce) can no-salt-added plum tomatoes

1 tablespoon olive oil

1 large onion, diced

8 ounces fresh mushrooms, sliced

1 (8-ounce) package organic tempeh, diced

3 cloves garlic, minced

1 teaspoon dried Italian seasoning

½ teaspoon freshly ground black pepper

⅛ teaspoon dried red pepper flakes

What Is Tempeh?

Tempeh is a fermented soybean product sold in firm rectangular cakes. It has a rugged texture and nutty flavor that melds well with many types of food. Cut it into cubes and add to pasta sauce, sauté along with vegetables, or marinate in your favorite sauce and bake. Tempeh is stocked in most supermarkets beside the tofu and refrigerated fake meat products. SoyBoy and Lightlife are two excellent brands. Tempeh is cholesterol free and a good source of protein, calcium, and iron.

1. Cook linguine according to package directions, omitting salt. Drain and set aside.

2. Chop the tomatoes and set aside with reserved juice from can.

3. Heat oil in a sauté pan over medium heat. Add the onion, mushrooms, tempeh, and garlic and cook, stirring, for 5 minutes.

4. Add the tomatoes with juice and seasonings. Cook, stirring occasionally, for 10 minutes.

5. Spoon sauce over pasta and serve immediately.

PER SERVING | Calories: 358 | Fat: 8 g | Protein: 19 g | Sodium: 27 mg | Fiber: 10 g | Carbohydrates: 60 g | Sugar: 5 g

Sweet Potatoes Stuffed with Chili

A quick and easy meatless meal made for improvisation. Use regular potatoes instead of sweet, add corn instead of peas, substitute kidney or pinto beans for black, plain yogurt for the sour cream, and so on. It's a meal that's adaptable, not to mention cheap and tasty, and without the sour cream, it's even vegan! Adapted from Prevention's Low-Fat, Low-Cost Freezer Cookbook.

INGREDIENTS | SERVES 4

4 medium sweet potatoes

2 (15-ounce) cans no-salt-added black beans

¼ cup unsweetened apple juice

1 teaspoon olive oil

1 medium onion, diced

2 cloves garlic, minced

2 medium carrots, sliced

¼ cup low-sodium salsa

1 (14-ounce) can no-salt-added diced tomatoes

½ cup frozen peas

1 tablespoon salt-free chili seasoning

1 teaspoon ground cumin

Freshly ground black pepper, to taste

½ cup nonfat sour cream, optional

1. Scrub the sweet potatoes and pierce all over with the tines of a fork. Place potatoes on a paper towel and/or microwave-safe plate and microwave on high for 7 minutes. Turn potatoes over, then microwave for another 7 minutes.

2. Drain and rinse the black beans and set aside.

3. Combine the apple juice and oil in a sauté pan and bring to a boil over medium heat. Add the onion and garlic and cook, stirring, for 3 minutes.

4. Add the carrots and salsa and sauté until softened, about 5 minutes.

5. Add the beans, tomatoes with juice, peas, and seasonings. Reduce heat to low, cover, and cook, stirring frequently, for 20 minutes.

6. Carefully split each sweet potato open and mash slightly. Spoon a quarter of the chili over each sweet potato and top with a dollop of sour cream if desired. Serve immediately.

PER SERVING | Calories: 493 | Fat: 2 g | Protein: 23 g | Sodium: 162 mg | Fiber: 18 g | Carbohydrates: 99 g | Sugar: 20 g

Coconut Cauliflower Curry

Coconut milk, vegetable broth, garlic, and ginger. This intoxicating array of flavors and more make this a heavenly vegetarian meal. If you don't have garam masala, substitute salt-free curry powder instead. Serve with steamed brown or basmati rice.

INGREDIENTS | SERVES 6

1 tablespoon canola oil

1 medium onion, diced

6 cloves garlic, minced

1 tablespoon minced fresh ginger

1 tablespoon salt-free garam masala

1 teaspoon ground turmeric

2 tablespoons salt-free tomato paste

2 cups low-sodium vegetable broth

1 cup light coconut milk

1 head cauliflower, cut into florets

3 medium potatoes or sweet potatoes, diced

2 medium carrots, sliced

1 (15-ounce) can no-salt-added diced tomatoes

1½ cups fresh or frozen peas

½ teaspoon freshly ground black pepper

¼ cup chopped fresh cilantro

1. Heat oil in a stockpot over medium heat. Add onion, garlic, and ginger and cook, stirring, for 5 minutes.

2. Add the garam masala and turmeric and sauté until fragrant, roughly 30 seconds to 1 minute.

3. Stir in the tomato paste, broth, coconut milk, cauliflower, potatoes, carrots, and tomatoes with juice and stir well to combine. Raise heat slightly and bring to a boil. Once boiling, lower heat to medium-low, cover, and simmer for 20 minutes.

4. Stir in the peas and black pepper and cook 2–3 minutes more.

5. Remove from heat and stir in the cilantro. Serve immediately.

PER SERVING | Calories: 178 | Fat: 6 g | Protein: 5 g | Sodium: 117 mg | Fiber: 7 g | Carbohydrates: 27 g | Sugar: 11 g

What Is Garam Masala?

Garam masala is a ground spice blend used extensively in Indian cooking. Though blends may differ, garam masala typically includes cinnamon, cumin, coriander, cloves, ginger, nutmeg, pepper, mace, star anise, and/or bay leaves. Garam masala is potent in terms of fragrance and flavor, but unlike many curry powders does not tend to be fiery hot.

Spicy Red Lentil Dal with Vegetables

This filling main course is a snap to prepare and sings with the mingling flavors of ginger, garlic, and cilantro. If you prefer less spice, simply omit the chili pepper. Be sure to prep all the ingredients beforehand for ease. Serve over cooked rice, sprinkled with additional cilantro, if desired. Adapted from Fine Cooking.

INGREDIENTS | SERVES 6

1 medium onion, diced

4 cloves garlic, minced

2 tablespoons minced fresh ginger

1 hot pepper, your choice

2 teaspoons canola oil

1½ teaspoons mustard seeds

1 tablespoon salt-free garam masala or curry powder

1½ cups red lentils, rinsed well

½ head cauliflower, broken into florets

4 medium carrots, cut into 1-inch pieces

2 large potatoes, cut into 1-inch chunks

1 teaspoon ground turmeric

6 cups water

¾ cup chopped fresh cilantro

Freshly ground black pepper, to taste

1. Place the onion, garlic, ginger, and hot pepper into a food processor and pulse briefly to chop.

2. Heat the oil in a stockpot over medium heat. When hot, add the mustard seeds. When the seeds begin to pop, stir in the garam masala or curry powder, onion mixture, lentils, cauliflower, carrots, potatoes, turmeric, and water.

3. Raise heat slightly and bring to a boil. Once boiling, reduce heat to medium-low, cover, and simmer until vegetables are tender, about 20–25 minutes.

4. Stir in the cilantro and season to taste with freshly ground black pepper. Serve immediately.

PER SERVING | Calories: 198 | Fat: 2 g | Protein: 11 g | Sodium: 39 mg | Fiber: 10 g | Carbohydrates: 35 g | Sugar: 5 g

Tofu and Veggie Stir-Fry

A delicious meal in minutes, packed with fresh taste and healthful ingredients.
Serve over cooked brown rice.

INGREDIENTS | SERVES 4

1 pound extra-firm tofu

2 teaspoons sesame oil

1 bunch broccoli, cut into florets

1 head bok choy, chopped

3 medium carrots, sliced

1 cup fresh pea pods

3 scallions, sliced

3 cloves garlic, minced

1 tablespoon minced fresh ginger

2 teaspoons low-sodium soy sauce

½ teaspoon ground white pepper

2 tablespoons water

1. Drain tofu and gently press between paper towels to release as much liquid as possible. Cut into 1-inch cubes and set aside.

2. Heat oil in a wok over medium-high heat. Add vegetables, garlic, ginger, soy sauce, and white pepper and stir-fry for 3 minutes.

3. Add water and tofu and stir-fry for another 3 minutes.

4. Remove from heat and serve immediately.

PER SERVING | Calories: 206 | Fat: 9 g | Protein: 16 g | Sodium: 184 mg | Fiber: 5 g | Carbohydrates: 18 g | Sugar: 7 g

The Soy Sauce Dilemma

The salty flavor of soy sauce makes many Asian dishes distinctively delicious, but traditional soy sauce is prohibitively high in sodium. Nonvegetarians may substitute Faux Soy Sauce instead (see Chapter 5). But if you're looking for a vegetarian alternative, what to use? Low-sodium soy sauce is sold in many supermarkets and online; House of Tsang or San-J are two of the lowest-sodium brands. Bragg Liquid Aminos and Coconut Secret Coconut Aminos are also good soy sauce replacements and are sold at Whole Foods, select stores, and online.

CHAPTER 14

Sandwiches

Black Bean Burgers

Southwestern flavor in a hearty veggie burger.
Garnish with homemade guacamole and salsa.

INGREDIENTS | SERVES 4

2 (15-ounce) cans no-salt-added black beans
1 shallot, minced
3 cloves garlic, minced
1 medium red bell pepper, chopped
¼ cup chopped fresh cilantro
1 tablespoon freshly squeezed lime juice
2 teaspoons salt-free chili seasoning
Freshly ground black pepper, to taste
½ cup salt-free bread crumbs

1. Preheat oven to 425°F. Spray a baking sheet lightly with oil and set aside.

2. Drain and rinse the beans, then place in a food processor and purée until smooth.

3. Transfer the beans to a mixing bowl, add remaining ingredients, and mix together using your (freshly washed) hands. Form into 4 large patties.

4. Place patties on prepared baking sheet. Place baking sheet on middle rack in oven and bake for 10 minutes. Remove from oven, gently flip, and return patties to oven. Bake for another 5 minutes.

5. Remove from oven and serve immediately.

PER SERVING (1 PATTY) | Calories: 348 | Fat: 1 g | Protein: 19 g | Sodium: 11 mg | Fiber: 13 g | Carbohydrates: 69 g | Sugar: 3 g

Seasoned Turkey Burgers
with Sautéed Mushrooms and Swiss

*These juicy, salt-free burgers will have you oohing and ahhing
your way to the last mushroom-topped bite.*

INGREDIENTS | SERVES 4

1 pound lean ground turkey

2 cloves garlic, minced

1 tablespoon salt-free prepared mustard

2 teaspoons low-sodium Worcestershire sauce

1 teaspoon dried Italian seasoning

½ teaspoon freshly ground black pepper

1 teaspoon olive oil

3 cups sliced mushrooms

4 Soft and Crusty No-Rise Sandwich Rolls (see Chapter 3)

½ cup shredded Swiss cheese

An Easy Way to Clean Your Grill

Whether you own a charcoal or propane grill, the easiest way to clean it is right after use. After removing food from the grill, close the lid, and allow the flames to burn off excess grease and debris. After about 10 minutes, go back and scrape the grates with a heavy wire brush. Turn off the gas (if applicable) and close the lid again. The grill is now ready for your next cookout.

1. Place the ground turkey into a mixing bowl. Add the garlic, mustard, Worcestershire sauce, Italian seasoning, and black pepper and mix well using your (freshly washed) hands. Divide mixture into 4 equal parts. Roll each portion into a round ball, then flatten and form into patties.

2. Grill or broil the burgers until they reach an internal temperature of 165°F. If grilling, roughly 5–6 minutes per side; if broiling, 4–6 minutes per side. Remove burgers from heat, cover, and set aside.

3. Heat the oil in a sauté pan over medium heat. Add the mushrooms and cook, stirring, for 5 minutes. Remove from heat.

4. Sandwich each burger in a bun, dividing sautéed mushrooms and cheese evenly among them. Serve immediately.

PER SERVING | Calories: 377 | Fat: 14 g | Protein: 32 g | Sodium: 145 mg | Fiber: 3 g | Carbohydrates: 31 g | Sugar: 3 g

Spinach Burgers

A different way to enjoy your spinach, these burgers are thick, meaty, and completely vegetarian. The shredded Swiss cheese adds a melty tang while keeping the sodium low. Cooked quinoa may be substituted for the salt-free bread crumbs for delicious gluten-free burgers.

INGREDIENTS | SERVES 4

1 teaspoon olive oil
1 medium red onion, diced
4 cloves garlic, minced
1 medium red bell pepper, diced
6 cups fresh baby spinach
1½ teaspoons dried Italian seasoning
½ teaspoon freshly ground black pepper
1 egg white
¼ cup shredded Swiss cheese
½ cup salt-free bread crumbs

1. Preheat oven to 425°F. Spray a baking sheet lightly with oil and set aside.

2. Heat oil in a sauté pan over medium heat. Add the onion and garlic and sauté for 2 minutes.

3. Add bell pepper and sauté for 2 minutes.

4. Add the spinach and sauté until wilted, about 2 minutes more. Remove pan from heat.

5. Add seasonings and stir well, scraping up the brown bits from the bottom of the pan. Set aside to cool for 5 minutes.

6. Add egg white, cheese, and bread crumbs to pan and stir well to combine. Form mixture into 4 patties.

7. Remove pan from heat. Place patties on prepared baking sheet. Place sheet on middle rack in oven and bake for 10 minutes. Flip patties and bake for another 5 minutes.

8. Remove from oven and serve immediately.

PER SERVING | Calories: 111 | Fat: 3 g | Protein: 6 g | Sodium: 66 mg | Fiber: 2 g | Carbohydrates: 15 g | Sugar: 1 g

Salmon Cakes

Thanks to Healthy Heart Market, Trader Joe's, Whole Foods Market, and others, you can buy canned salt-free salmon without difficulty or tremendous expense. Delicately crisp outside and flavorfully moist inside, these salmon cakes are a real treat whether sandwiched in rolls or eaten plain.

INGREDIENTS | SERVES 6

1 (15-ounce) can no-salt-added boneless salmon

4 tablespoons Salt-Free Mayonnaise (see Chapter 5)

½ cup salt-free bread crumbs

1 small onion, chopped finely

1 small bell pepper, chopped finely

1 egg white

1 teaspoon dried herbes de Provence

½ teaspoon ground sweet paprika

¼ teaspoon dry ground mustard

⅛ teaspoon celery seed

Freshly ground black pepper, to taste

Mayonnaise Substitute

Instead of adding salt-free mayonnaise to a recipe, try substituting an equal amount of plain nonfat Greek yogurt. Its thick and creamy consistency works well in many types of salads and sandwiches, from tuna and salmon to chicken and egg. To thin the yogurt, add a little lemon juice or low-sodium broth. For added flavor, add minced garlic and some chopped fresh herbs.

1. Preheat oven to 400°F. Spray a baking sheet lightly with oil and set aside.

2. Drain salmon well and place into a mixing bowl. Add remaining ingredients and mix well using a spoon or your (freshly washed) hands. Divide mixture into 6 equal portions and shape into patties.

3. Place patties on the prepared baking sheet. Place baking sheet on middle rack in oven and bake for 10 minutes. Remove from oven, gently flip, and return to oven to bake 5 minutes more.

4. Remove from oven and serve immediately.

PER SERVING | Calories: 202 | Fat: 11 g | Protein: 16 g | Sodium: 68 mg | Fiber: 1 g | Carbohydrates: 8 g | Sugar: 1 g

Portabella Burgers

One of the simplest and best burgers ever. Grilled portabella mushrooms are so naturally juicy and meaty you may swear off hamburgers forever.

INGREDIENTS | SERVES 4

4 large portabella mushroom caps

1 tablespoon olive oil

4 Soft and Crusty No-Rise Sandwich Rolls (See Chapter 3)

1. Preheat grill.

2. Brush mushroom caps with oil. Place flat side on grill and cook for 8 minutes. Flip mushrooms over and grill another 5 minutes.

3. Remove mushrooms from grill and sandwich between rolls. Garnish with condiments of choice. Serve immediately.

PER SERVING | Calories: 201 | Fat: 5 g | Protein: 7 g | Sodium: 14 mg | Fiber: 4 g | Carbohydrates: 32 g | Sugar: 3 g

Ground Turkey Sloppy Joes

Tangy, sweet, and slightly sour, these sloppy joes are every bit as good as the salty ones you used to enjoy.

INGREDIENTS | SERVES 4

1 pound lean ground turkey

1 medium onion, diced

3 cloves garlic, minced

1 medium red bell pepper, diced

1 medium tomato, diced

1 (8-ounce) can no-salt-added tomato sauce

1 (6-ounce) can salt-free tomato paste

¼ cup apple cider vinegar

2 tablespoons brown sugar

1 teaspoon dried oregano

½ teaspoon ground cumin

Freshly ground black pepper, to taste

4 Soft and Crusty No-Rise Sandwich Rolls (see Chapter 3)

1. Place the ground turkey, onion, and garlic in a sauté pan over medium heat. Cook, stirring, for 5 minutes.

2. Add remaining ingredients and stir to combine. Reduce heat to medium-low and simmer for 20 minutes, stirring occasionally. Remove from heat.

3. Divide mixture evenly between rolls. Serve immediately.

PER SERVING | Calories: 407 | Fat: 9 g | Protein: 30 g | Sodium: 142 mg | Fiber: 6 g | Carbohydrates: 52 g | Sugar: 18 g

Grilled Chicken Patties

Lean ground chicken plus Southwestern spice makes one yummy burger. And they're so low in sodium, you can splurge and sandwich them between regular whole-grain buns!

INGREDIENTS | SERVES 4

1 pound lean ground chicken
1 teaspoon ground sweet paprika
½ teaspoon freshly ground black pepper
½ teaspoon ground cumin
½ teaspoon salt-free chili seasoning
¼ teaspoon dried red pepper flakes

Keeping Grilled Burgers Juicy

Burgers have a tendency to round upward while cooking on the grill. To keep patties flat while cooking, make a small indentation in the center of each side using the back of a spoon or your thumb. The indented centers will rise to meet the rest of the burger, without the need for flattening. Grilled burgers will remain juicy and delicious.

1. Preheat grill.

2. Place ground chicken into a mixing bowl. Add the seasonings and mix thoroughly using your (freshly washed) hands. Divide mixture into 4 equal portions. Roll each portion into a ball, then flatten to form patties.

3. Once grill is ready, place patties on surface. Grill for 5–6 minutes on the first side, then gently flip patties and grill for another 5–6 minutes on the second side.

4. Remove from grill, place on buns if desired, and serve immediately.

PER SERVING | Calories: 118 | Fat: 2 g | Protein: 20 g | Sodium: 73 mg | Fiber: 0 g | Carbohydrates: 1 g | Sugar: 0 g

Tropical Chicken Salad Wrap Sandwiches

Colorfully festive with a fresh, spicy kick, these sandwiches make great party fare sliced in half and arranged on a platter. The filling eschews mayo in favor of a light vinaigrette. Serve with sliced avocado if desired. Garden City Brand All Natural Lavash Roll-Ups are available at Whole Foods markets.

INGREDIENTS | SERVES 6

1 pound boneless, skinless chicken breasts
1 ripe mango, diced
1 small red onion, diced
1 small bell pepper, diced
1 jalapeño pepper, minced
2 cloves garlic, minced
1 cup cooked no-salt-added black beans
2 tablespoons apple cider vinegar
Juice of 1 freshly squeezed lime
2 tablespoons olive oil
¼ cup chopped fresh cilantro
½ teaspoon ground white pepper
4 cups mixed salad greens
1 package Garden City Brand All Natural Square Lavash

1. Place chicken breasts into a pot and add enough water to cover. Bring to a boil over high heat. Once boiling, reduce heat slightly and continue boiling about 20 minutes, until fully cooked. Remove from heat, drain, and set aside to cool.

2. Once cool to touch, cut chicken into bite-sized pieces. Place into a mixing bowl and add the mango, onion, peppers, garlic, and beans.

3. Place the vinegar, lime juice, oil, cilantro, and pepper into a small bowl and whisk well to combine. Pour over the chicken salad and stir well to coat.

4. Divide greens and chicken salad evenly between the lavash, then roll the sandwiches up. Slice each sandwich in half using a sharp knife.

5. Serve immediately or cover and refrigerate until serving.

PER SERVING | Calories: 369 | Fat: 10 g | Protein: 30 g | Sodium: 77 mg | Fiber: 4 g | Carbohydrates: 45 g | Sugar: 6 g

Open-Faced Tuna Melts

This lightened version of the beloved diner sandwich uses homemade salt-free mayo, leaving the sandwiches lower in both fat and cholesterol.

INGREDIENTS | SERVES 2

1 (5-ounce) can no-salt-added tuna in water

1 shallot, finely chopped

1 small stalk celery, finely diced

1 small carrot, finely diced

2 tablespoons Salt-Free Mayonnaise (see Chapter 5)

¼ cup chopped Sweet and Spicy Salt-Free Pickles (see Chapter 2) with brine

½ teaspoon dried herbes de Provence

Freshly ground black pepper, to taste

2 slices low-sodium bread

2 slices romaine lettuce

1 small ripe tomato, sliced

2 slices Swiss cheese

1. Preheat the broiler. Take out a baking sheet and set aside.

2. Drain the tuna and place into a mixing bowl. Add the shallot, celery, carrot, mayonnaise, chopped pickles, and herbes de Provence and stir well to combine. Season with freshly ground black pepper, to taste.

3. Place the 2 slices of bread on the baking sheet. Top each with a lettuce slice, then divide the tuna mixture between the two and smooth to even. Top with sliced tomato and cheese.

4. Place baking sheet on top rack in oven and broil for 1–2 minutes, until cheese has melted completely. Remove from oven and serve immediately.

PER SERVING | Calories: 368 | Fat: 18 g | Protein: 29 g | Sodium: 130 mg | Fiber: 1 g | Carbohydrates: 21 g | Sugar: 4 g

Herbes de Provence

A classic blend of French herbs, typically comprised of dried basil, thyme, savory, fennel, and lavender, herbes de Provence gives a distinct flavor to many dishes and is particularly well suited to grilled meats and seafood. Commercial blends are sold in supermarkets and online.

Egg Salad Sandwiches with Radish and Cilantro

Creamy eggs contrast with the spicy bite of the radish, pungent cilantro, and a subtle rice vinegar tang. It's a seemingly incongruous combination of flavors that works so well together.

INGREDIENTS | SERVES 4

6 eggs
1 cup shredded radish
¼ cup chopped fresh cilantro
1 tablespoon olive oil
1 tablespoon unflavored rice vinegar
¼ teaspoon freshly ground black pepper
2 cups arugula
8 slices whole-grain salt-free bread

1. Place eggs into a saucepan and add enough water to cover by 1 or 2 inches. Place pan over high heat and bring to a boil. Simmer for 12 minutes. Remove from heat and place under cold running water. When eggs are cool enough to handle, gently crack, peel, and dice. Place into a medium bowl.

2. Add shredded radish, cilantro, oil, vinegar, and pepper and stir well to combine.

3. Assemble the sandwiches by dividing the arugula and egg salad evenly between 4 slices of bread. Top each with another slice. Serve immediately.

PER SERVING | Calories: 287 | Fat: 13 g | Protein: 14 g | Sodium: 120 mg | Fiber: 4 g | Carbohydrates: 27 g | Sugar: 4 g

Roasted Red Pepper Hummus, Carrot, and Parsley Wrap Sandwiches

The perfect sandwich for a hot summer day. Cool, refreshing, and supremely healthy, these vegan wraps satisfy hunger without weighing you down. Add additional veggies or lettuce as desired.

INGREDIENTS | SERVES 4

1 package Garden City Brand All Natural Square Lavash

1 cup Roasted Red Pepper Hummus (see Chapter 5)

2 medium carrots, shredded

½ cup chopped fresh parsley

Flavor Your Hummus

When you tire of garlic or red pepper hummus, try making some of these. Stir the juice and grated zest of a large fresh lemon into plain hummus for a citrus splash. For a spicy Southwestern hummus, add lime juice, minced jalapeño, ground cumin, and a little salt-free chili seasoning. Ground 5-spice powder, minced fresh ginger, and scallions make a tasty Asian-style hummus. Or create a veggie-centric hummus by adding puréed sautéed vegetables and a little low-sodium broth.

1. Spread the lavash on a clean surface.

2. Measure ¼ cup hummus onto the center of each wrap and spread to even. Top with a quarter of the shredded carrot and parsley.

3. Fold the top and bottom of the lavash toward the filling, fold one of the sides over the filling to cover, and then carefully roll to close. Repeat with remaining sandwiches. Serve immediately.

PER SERVING | Calories: 384 | Fat: 8 g | Protein: 5 g | Sodium: 72 mg | Fiber: 8 g | Carbohydrates: 71 g | Sugar: 6 g

Barbecued Tempeh Sandwiches

A quick and tasty meal as filling as it is flavorful. The tempeh mixture is also delicious spooned over rice, couscous, or baked potatoes.

INGREDIENTS | SERVES 6

2 teaspoons olive oil

1 (8-ounce) package organic tempeh, diced

1 large onion, diced

1 medium bell pepper, diced

3 cloves garlic, minced

1 (15-ounce) can no-salt-added diced tomatoes

2 (8-ounce) cans no-salt-added tomato sauce

1 tablespoon apple cider vinegar

1 tablespoon molasses

1½ teaspoons low-sodium Worcestershire sauce

1 teaspoon ground sweet paprika

½ teaspoon freshly ground black pepper

½ teaspoon ground cumin

¼ teaspoon ground cinnamon

¼ teaspoon liquid smoke

⅛ teaspoon ground cayenne pepper

¼ cup chopped fresh cilantro

6 Soft and Crusty No-Rise Sandwich Rolls (see Chapter 3)

1. Heat oil in a sauté pan over medium heat. Add tempeh, onion, bell pepper, and garlic and sauté for 5 minutes.

2. Add remaining ingredients except for the cilantro, reduce heat to medium-low, and cook for another 15 minutes, stirring frequently. Remove from heat.

3. Stir in cilantro and spoon tempeh mixture into buns. Serve immediately.

PER SERVING | Calories: 297 | Fat: 8 g | Protein: 14 g | Sodium: 44 mg | Fiber: 5 g | Carbohydrates: 45 g | Sugar: 10 g

Tofu Sloppy Joes

If you're skeptical of tofu, give this recipe a try. Freezing and thawing the tofu changes its texture, giving it a much meatier feel. Add sautéed veggies, tomato sauce, and a vinegar tang, and it's absolutely transformed. Adapted from The Healthy Cook.

INGREDIENTS | SERVES 4

1 pound extra-firm tofu, frozen and thawed

2 teaspoons canola oil

1 medium onion, diced

1 medium bell pepper, diced

1 medium stalk celery, diced

2 (8-ounce) cans no-salt-added tomato sauce

1½ tablespoons apple cider vinegar

1 tablespoon salt-free prepared mustard

¾ teaspoon low-sodium Worcestershire sauce

1 teaspoon sugar

Freshly ground black pepper, to taste

4 Soft and Crusty No-Rise Sandwich Rolls (See Chapter 3)

1. Drain tofu and press firmly between 2 plates to release any additional liquid. Pat dry with paper towels, then crumble the tofu coarsely with a fork or your fingers.

2. Heat the oil in a sauté pan over medium heat. Add the tofu, onions, green pepper, and celery and sauté for 8 minutes.

3. Stir in the tomato sauce, vinegar, mustard, Worcestershire sauce, and sugar. Cook, stirring frequently, for 5 minutes.

4. Remove from heat and season to taste with freshly ground black pepper. Divide the mixture evenly between the buns. Serve immediately.

PER SERVING | Calories: 348 | Fat: 1 g | Protein: 18 g | Sodium: 46 mg | Fiber: 6 g | Carbohydrates: 45 g | Sugar: 10 g

Versatile Tofu

Tofu soaks up flavors like nothing else, and can be added to almost any type of dish, providing added protein, calcium, and iron. Cube a pound of extra-firm tofu, add to assorted vegetables, and roast. Slice into sticks, bake, and toss with a little nutritional yeast. Crumble and add to a veggie stir-fry with brown rice. Or use instead of chicken in a vegetarian noodle soup.

Beef and Bean Burritos

These hearty meal-size burritos are so tasty, you'll hardly believe they're low sodium. Store any leftover filling in the fridge and it'll be as good or even better the next day. If you run out of lavash, simply warm the filling and serve alongside salsa, sour cream, and unsalted tortilla chips for a delicious new take on nachos.

INGREDIENTS | SERVES 4

1 pound extra-lean ground beef

1 medium onion, diced finely

1 jalapeño pepper, minced

2 cloves garlic, minced

1 (15-ounce) can no-salt-added black beans

⅔ cup fresh or frozen corn kernels

1 tablespoon salt-free tomato ketchup

1 tablespoon salt-free tomato paste

1 teaspoon honey

¾ teaspoon liquid smoke

1½ teaspoons ground cumin

1 teaspoon ground sweet paprika

½ teaspoon ground coriander

½ teaspoon ground mustard

1 package Garden City Brand All Natural Square Lavash

1 cup low-sodium tomato salsa

½ cup nonfat sour cream

¼ cup chopped fresh cilantro

1. Brown the ground beef in a skillet or sauté pan over medium heat. Add the onion, jalapeño, and garlic and sauté for 5 minutes.

2. Drain the black beans and add to the pan, along with the corn, ketchup, tomato paste, honey, liquid smoke, and seasonings. Reduce heat to medium-low and cook for 10 minutes, stirring frequently. Remove from heat.

3. Place the lavash on a clean surface and divide filling evenly between them. Top each with 3 tablespoons salsa, 1½ tablespoons sour cream, and 1 tablespoon chopped cilantro.

4. Fold the top and bottom of the roll-up toward the filling, fold one of the sides over the filling to cover, and then carefully roll to close. Repeat with remaining burritos. Serve immediately.

PER SERVING | Calories: 605 | Fat: 10 g | Protein: 42 g | Sodium: 285 mg | Fiber: 8 g | Carbohydrates: 94 g | Sugar: 11 g

Cut the Fat

When choosing ground beef or other meats, always buy the leanest cuts possible. When you compare fat for a 4-ounce serving of ground beef, for instance, you can cut your fat intake in half simply by opting for the slightly more expensive 95 percent lean (5.6 g fat) over the 90 percent lean (11 g fat). Leaner meat may be more expensive, but better health is worth the small investment.

Sweet Potato and Black Bean Burritos

The perfect quick meal, from stovetop to table in 30 minutes. The filling is an irresistible combination of flavors and textures, both sweet and savory. Dotted with luscious nonfat sour cream, spicy salsa, and the bite of cilantro, it's perfect. Spoon into low-sodium taco shells if you can't find lavash. Adapted from Simply in Season.

INGREDIENTS | SERVES 4

3 small–medium sweet potatoes

1 tablespoon canola oil

1 medium onion, diced

¾ cup unsweetened apple juice

1 (15 ounce) can no-salt-added black beans

1 teaspoon ground cumin

½ teaspoon ground cinnamon

½ teaspoon salt-free chili seasoning

Freshly ground black pepper, to taste

1 package Garden City Brand All Natural Square Lavash

¼ cup low-sodium salsa

¼ cup nonfat sour cream

¼ cup chopped fresh cilantro

1. Peel the sweet potatoes and cut into ½-inch cubes.

2. Heat the oil in a sauté pan over medium heat. Add the diced sweet potato, onion, and ½ cup apple juice to the pan and stir to combine. Cover the pan and cook, stirring frequently, until sweet potatoes are tender, about 20 minutes.

3. Drain the black beans. Uncover the pan and add the beans, the remaining apple juice, and seasonings and stir to combine. Cook, stirring, for 5 minutes. Remove pan from heat.

4. Place the lavash on a clean surface. Top each with ¼ of the burrito mixture, salsa, sour cream, and cilantro.

5. Fold ends toward the center, then roll from the other side up into a cylinder. Slice burritos in half using a sharp knife. Serve immediately.

PER SERVING | Calories: 470 | Fat: 8 g | Protein: 18 g | Sodium: 112 mg | Fiber: 9 g | Carbohydrates: 90 g | Sugar: 9 g

Vegetarian Refried Bean Burritos

*These yummy, guilt-free burritos whip together in minutes,
making them a great go-to meal anytime.*

INGREDIENTS | SERVES 4

2 (15-ounce) cans no-salt-added pinto beans

2 teaspoons canola oil

1 medium onion, finely diced

3 cloves garlic, minced

¼ cup low-sodium vegetable broth

Juice of 1 fresh lime

1 teaspoon ground cumin

½ teaspoon ground coriander

¾ teaspoon freshly ground black pepper

1 package Garden City Brand All Natural Square Lavash

Pinto Bean Facts

Pinto in Spanish means "painted," which describes the speckled exterior of these tasty and nutritious beans. High in protein, folate, fiber, and minerals, pinto beans are an excellent addition to a healthy diet. Add them to chilis, soups and salads, layer with vegetables and bake for a hot casserole, or mash to make a dip or sandwich spread.

1. Drain beans, place in a food processor, and purée.

2. Heat oil in a sauté pan over medium heat. Add onion and garlic and cook, stirring, for 3 minutes.

3. Reduce heat to medium-low, add puréed beans, broth, lime juice, and seasonings and cook, stirring, for 2 minutes. Add additional broth to thin as desired. Remove from heat.

4. Place the lavash on a clean surface. Top each with ¼ of the refried beans. Fold ends toward the center, then roll up into a cylinder. Serve immediately.

PER SERVING | Calories: 586 | Fat: 7 g | Protein: 27 g | Sodium: 225 mg | Fiber: 20 g | Carbohydrates: 112 g | Sugar: <1 g

Falafel with Tzatziki

These little vegetarian chickpea patties are such a nice change from the everyday, they'll feel like a special treat. Wrap in low-sodium pita or lavash or enjoy plain.

INGREDIENTS | SERVES 4

1 (15-ounce) can no-salt-added garbanzo beans
1 small onion
3 cloves garlic
¼ cup fresh parsley
2 teaspoons ground cumin
1 teaspoon ground coriander
¼ teaspoon dried red pepper flakes
Freshly ground black pepper, to taste
1 small cucumber
2 cloves garlic, finely minced
1 tablespoon chopped fresh dill
1 teaspoon freshly squeezed lemon juice
¾ cup plain nonfat Greek yogurt
Ground white pepper, to taste

1. Preheat the oven to 400°F. Spray a baking sheet lightly with oil and set aside.

2. Drain and rinse the chickpeas, then place into a food processor. Add the onion, 3 cloves garlic, parsley, cumin, coriander, red pepper flakes, and freshly ground black pepper to taste. Pulse until smooth.

3. Spoon by large tablespoonfuls onto the prepared baking sheet. Place sheet on middle rack in oven and bake for 10 minutes. Remove from oven, gently flip falafel patties, and return to bake for another 5–10 minutes.

4. While falafel is baking, peel the cucumber. Slice lengthwise and gently scrape out seeds using a spoon. Grate, then place into a clean towel and squeeze to remove excess liquid.

5. Place into a mixing bowl and add the remaining ingredients. Season to taste with ground white pepper and stir well to combine.

6. Remove falafel from oven and serve immediately with tzatziki.

PER SERVING | Calories: 195 | Fat: 3 g | Protein: 11 g | Sodium: 15 mg | Fiber: 8 g | Carbohydrates: 22 g | Sugar: 6 g

Meatless Meatball Sandwiches

These vegetarian meatballs look and taste so authentic, you'll have difficulty telling the difference. Serve in buns with salt-free marinara sauce or spooned over pasta. Adapted from the American Heart Association's Recipes for the Heart.

INGREDIENTS | SERVES 6

½ cup low-sodium vegetable broth

⅓ cup dry bulgur

1 teaspoon olive oil

1 cup chopped fresh mushrooms

3 scallions, sliced

1 tablespoon balsamic vinegar

⅓ cup chopped walnuts

⅓ cup salt-free bread crumbs

1 egg

2 egg whites

½ teaspoon dried thyme

¼ teaspoon dried red pepper flakes

1 (25-ounce) jar salt-free pasta sauce

6 low-sodium sandwich rolls

Baked Meatballs

Many types of meatballs may be oven baked instead of pan fried or simmered. Shape meatball mixture into 2-inch balls and place on a lightly oiled baking sheet. Bake at 400°F for roughly 20 minutes. White meats, such as chicken and turkey, tend to cook more quickly than red meats and may dry out if overbaked, so watch carefully. Meatballs are done when they're no longer pink inside.

1. Measure the broth and bulgur into a small saucepan and stir to combine. Bring to a boil over high heat. Once boiling, reduce heat to low, cover, and simmer for 10 minutes. Drain any excess broth and set aside.

2. Heat oil in a sauté pan over medium heat. Add the mushrooms and scallions and cook, stirring, for 5 minutes. Stir in the vinegar. Remove from heat and spread mixture on a plate to cool to room temperature.

3. Once cool, place the mushroom mixture and walnuts into a food processor and pulse to chop. Add the bulgur and chop. Add the bread crumbs, egg, egg whites, thyme, and red pepper flakes and pulse to combine. Let stand for 5 minutes to absorb liquid.

4. Pour the pasta sauce into a sauté pan over medium heat and bring to a simmer. Once simmering, use a tablespoon to scoop out the meatball batter and gently add the meatballs to the pan. Reduce heat to low, cover, and simmer for 10–15 minutes, until the balls are firm. Turn the meatballs halfway through the cooking time, being very gentle so as not to break them.

5. Remove from heat and spoon into buns. Serve immediately.

PER SERVING | Calories: 313 | Fat: 8 g | Protein: 11 g | Sodium: 65 mg | Fiber: 6 g | Carbohydrates: 50 g | Sugar: 9 g

CHAPTER 15

Side Dishes

Lemon Parmesan Rice with Fresh Herbs

A healthy, quick, and easy side with lots of flavor. Vary the fresh herbs to suit your mood;
it's particularly tasty with parsley, cilantro, or basil.

INGREDIENTS | SERVES 4

1 cup basmati rice

1½ cups low-sodium chicken or vegetable broth

2 tablespoons grated Parmesan cheese

2 tablespoons chopped fresh herbs

1 tablespoon freshly squeezed lemon juice

½ teaspoon grated lemon zest

½ teaspoon freshly ground black pepper

1. Rinse rice well in a fine-mesh sieve, then place in a saucepan.

2. Add broth and bring to a boil over medium-high heat. Once boiling, reduce heat to low, cover, and simmer for 15 minutes.

3. Remove pan from heat. Add remaining ingredients and stir gently to combine. Serve immediately.

PER SERVING | Calories: 172 | Fat: 2 g | Protein: 6 g | Sodium: 67 mg | Fiber: 1 g | Carbohydrates: 32 g | Sugar: 0 g

Braised Brussels Sprouts with Apricots and Toasted Walnuts

A speedy and flavorful side brimming over with vitamins, protein, and fiber.
Dried cranberries may be substituted for the apricots if desired.

INGREDIENTS | SERVES 4

¼ cup chopped walnuts

1 pound Brussels sprouts, halved

2 shallots, minced

½ cup low-sodium vegetable broth

⅓ cup diced dried apricots

¼ teaspoon freshly ground black pepper

1. Place a sauté pan over medium heat. Add walnuts and toast, stirring, 2–3 minutes. Remove from pan and set aside.

2. Return pan to heat. Add Brussels sprouts, shallots, and broth and stir to combine. Cover pan and simmer, stirring once or twice, for 8 minutes.

3. Remove from heat. Stir in apricots, toasted walnuts, and black pepper. Serve immediately.

PER SERVING | Calories: 120 | Fat: 5 g | Protein: 4 g | Sodium: 43 mg | Fiber: 4 g | Carbohydrates: 17 g | Sugar: 7 g

Roasted Root Veggies with Orange and Thyme

A beautiful vegetable medley with a bright color and taste.
Cut the vegetables into equal-sized pieces to ensure even cooking.

INGREDIENTS | SERVES 6

3 medium carrots

3 medium parsnips

2 medium sweet potatoes

3 tablespoons freshly squeezed orange juice

1 tablespoon olive oil

1 tablespoon fresh thyme or 1 teaspoon dried

Freshly ground black pepper, to taste

Thyme Time

Thyme is an easy-to-grow perennial herb. Its strong, distinct flavor makes it a great choice for many types of roasts, soups, and stews. When using fresh thyme, gently run your fingers along its woody stem, removing the leaves. Leaves may be added whole or chopped. If fresh thyme is not available, dried thyme is a good alternative.

1. Preheat oven to 450°F. Take out a sided baking sheet and set aside.

2. Peel vegetables and cut into 1-inch pieces. Place in a mixing bowl, add remaining ingredients, and toss well to coat.

3. Turn mixture out onto baking sheet and arrange vegetables in a single layer.

4. Place baking sheet on middle rack in oven and bake for 30 minutes.

5. Remove from oven and serve immediately.

PER SERVING | Calories: 123 | Fat: 2 g | Protein: 2 g | Sodium: 43 mg | Fiber: 5 g | Carbohydrates: 24 g | Sugar: 7 g

Sweet and Savory Kale with Tomatoes

The combination of subtle sweetness and tang is addictive and so healthy. Use garden-ripe tomatoes when available, salt-free canned tomatoes when not. Chop the kale into bite-sized pieces, along with stems, for added fiber. Adapted from Rawl.net.

INGREDIENTS | SERVES 6

1¼ cups low-sodium vegetable broth

1 medium onion, diced

3 cloves garlic, minced

2 tablespoons salt-free prepared mustard

1 teaspoon sugar

1 tablespoon apple cider vinegar

1 pound chopped fresh kale

1 cup diced tomatoes

Freshly ground black pepper, to taste

1. Place a large stockpot or sauté pan over medium heat. Add ¼ cup broth, onion, and garlic and sauté for 2 minutes.

2. Add the mustard, sugar, vinegar, and remaining broth and stir to combine.

3. Add the kale and tomatoes and stir to coat. Cover the pot and cook, stirring occasionally, for 10 minutes, until kale is tender.

4. Remove from heat and season with freshly ground black pepper, to taste. Serve immediately.

PER SERVING | Calories: 53 | Fat: <1 g | Protein: 2 g | Sodium: 63 mg | Fiber: 2 g | Carbohydrates: 10 g | Sugar: 1 g

Kale Facts

Kale is a member of the cabbage family, grows easily in many climates, and freezes well. Once viewed as a decorative garnish, kale is increasingly taking center stage on the dinner plate. Its high levels of antioxidants make it an effective tool in the fight against cancer and cardiovascular disease. Kale contains twice the recommended daily value of vitamin A per serving, making it a valuable aid against degenerative eye diseases.

Roasted Red Peppers

Roasted peppers are beautiful, delicious, and truly easy to prepare. Use them to add color, flavor, and interest to a variety of dishes, from a simple Swiss cheese and roast chicken sandwich to a vegetarian hummus wrap to a salad of mushroom, onion, and kale. The possibilities are endless.

INGREDIENTS | YIELDS 1½ CUPS

3 large red bell peppers

1. Preheat oven to 450°F. Take out a baking sheet and set aside.

2. Halve peppers lengthwise, then remove core and seeds.

3. Lightly spray baking sheet with oil and place peppers on the sheet, cut-side down. Place baking sheet on middle rack in oven and bake 20–25 minutes, until skins are bubbled and beginning to char.

4. Remove baking sheet from oven and place on wire rack to cool briefly. Once peppers are cool enough to handle, gently remove skins.

5. Use immediately or store in an airtight container and refrigerate until use. These freeze well for up to 3 months.

PER SERVING (PER ½ CUP) | Calories: 50 | Fat: 0 g | Protein: 1 g | Sodium: 6 mg | Fiber: 3 g | Carbohydrates: 9 g | Sugar: 6 g

Sticky Caramelized Sweet Potato Spears

Sweet potatoes tossed with a mixture of brown sugar and salt-free chili seasoning, then baked. The resulting spears are sticky sweet, spicy, and delicious.

INGREDIENTS | SERVES 4

3 medium sweet potatoes

2 tablespoons olive oil

¼ cup brown sugar

1 teaspoon ground cinnamon

½ teaspoon salt-free chili seasoning

¼ teaspoon ground cumin

¼ teaspoon ground sweet paprika

Sweet Potato Facts

Sweet potatoes are often overlooked as holiday fare, something to be enjoyed certain times of the year and forgotten about the rest. But sweet potatoes are a staple we should all be embracing. They're inexpensive and incredibly versatile, adapting to almost any type of cuisine. They're full of vitamins A and C and beta-carotene, and super low in sodium. When buying sweet potatoes, look for firm, orange flesh, free of soft spots or blemishes. At home, store them in a dark cabinet or drawer, never in the refrigerator.

1. Preheat oven to 425°F. Line a baking sheet with aluminum foil and set aside.

2. Peel the sweet potatoes and cut in half lengthwise. Cut the halves lengthwise into spear-like wedges. Place the wedges into a large mixing bowl, add the olive oil, and toss well to coat.

3. Add the brown sugar and spices into a small mixing bowl and whisk well to combine. Sprinkle the mixture over the wedges and toss to coat.

4. Place the wedges on the baking sheet. Place baking sheet on the middle rack in oven and bake for 20 minutes. Carefully turn wedges, then return to oven and bake until soft, about 10 minutes.

5. Remove from oven and serve immediately.

PER SERVING | Calories: 198 | Fat: 7 g | Protein: 1 g | Sodium: 35 mg | Fiber: 3 g | Carbohydrates: 33 g | Sugar: 19 g

Sautéed Spinach with Shallots and Garlic

A deliciously healthy side in less than 10 minutes. Baby spinach requires nothing more than a good rinsing. When using larger spinach leaves, wash well, remove tough stems, then chop coarsely.

INGREDIENTS | SERVES 2

1 teaspoon olive oil
1 large shallot, minced
2 cloves garlic, minced
6 cups fresh spinach, washed well
Freshly ground black pepper, to taste

1. Heat oil in a sauté pan over medium heat. Add the shallot and garlic and sauté for 2 minutes.

2. Add the spinach and sauté just until wilted, roughly 3–5 minutes. Remove from heat.

3. Season with freshly ground black pepper, to taste. Serve immediately.

PER SERVING | Calories: 52 | Fat: 2 g | Protein: 3 g | Sodium: 72 mg | Fiber: 2 g | Carbohydrates: 6 g | Sugar: 0 g

Roasted Potatoes and Broccoli

The combination of crisp, flaky potatoes and slightly smoky broccoli is so simple and so good. Peel and cube the broccoli stem and add along with the florets; less waste, more fiber and nutrients.

INGREDIENTS | SERVES 6

4 medium potatoes, cubed
1 head fresh broccoli
1 medium onion
1 tablespoon olive oil
1 teaspoon all-purpose salt-free seasoning
½ teaspoon garlic powder
½ teaspoon ground rosemary
¼ teaspoon freshly ground black pepper

1. Preheat oven to 425°F. Take out a sided baking sheet.

2. Place the potatoes into a mixing bowl.

3. Cut the broccoli into florets, peel and cube the remaining stem if desired, and add to the bowl. Add the remaining ingredients and toss well to coat.

4. Spread mixture in a single layer on the baking pan.

5. Place pan on middle rack in oven and bake for 30 minutes. Remove from oven and serve immediately.

PER SERVING | Calories: 153 | Fat: 2 g | Protein: 4 g | Sodium: 48 mg | Fiber: 5 g | Carbohydrates: 30 g | Sugar: 3 g

Mushroom Barley Pilaf with Fresh Green Beans

This quick, healthy, and filling side also makes a great vegetarian main course. Quick barley speeds cooking time, getting this to the table in just 20 minutes. Substitute an equal amount of sliced garlic scapes for the garlic and green beans when in season.

INGREDIENTS | SERVES 4

1 cup dry quick barley

2 cups boiling water

1 teaspoon olive oil

1 medium red onion, diced

4 cloves garlic, minced

8 ounces fresh mushrooms, sliced

1 cup fresh green beans, cut into 1-inch pieces

¼ teaspoon dried marjoram

¼ teaspoon dried thyme

¼ teaspoon freshly ground black pepper

What Is Barley?

Barley is a type of whole grain, with a chewy texture and slightly nutty taste. Regular pearled barley cooks in about 40 minutes; quick barley is parboiled, allowing it to cook in a quarter of the time. Most of the barley grown in the United States is destined for beverages rather than food. Fermented barley, also known as barley malt, is an important ingredient in beer making. Barley is cholesterol free, low in fat, and high in fiber.

1. Measure barley into a saucepan and stir in boiling water. Place over high heat and bring to a boil. Once boiling, reduce heat to low, cover, and simmer for 10 minutes. Drain excess water and set aside.

2. Heat oil in a sauté pan over medium heat. Add onion and garlic and sauté for 2 minutes.

3. Add mushrooms and green beans and sauté for 5 minutes.

4. Remove from heat. Stir in barley and seasonings. Serve immediately.

PER SERVING | Calories: 183 | Fat: 2 g | Protein: 5 g | Sodium: 8 mg | Fiber: 6 g | Carbohydrates: 38 g | Sugar: 2 g

Israeli Couscous with Sautéed Spinach, Bell Pepper, and Onion

Earthy flavors accented with a splash of citrus, this yummy side can be served either warm or cold.

INGREDIENTS | SERVES 6

1⅓ cup uncooked Israeli couscous

1¾ cups boiling water

1 teaspoon olive oil

3 cloves garlic, minced

1 medium red onion, diced

1 medium red bell pepper, diced

6 cups fresh baby spinach

¼ cup low-sodium chicken or vegetable broth

2 tablespoons freshly squeezed lemon juice

¼ teaspoon freshly ground black pepper

What Is Israeli Couscous?

Israeli couscous, also known as ptitim, is a type of small, round pasta made from wheat flour. It's similar to standard couscous, but much larger in diameter. Israeli couscous cooks quickly and is very versatile, making it a great alternative to rice and other grains. It's sold in supermarkets and specialty food stores in both white and whole-wheat varieties.

1. Measure couscous into a saucepan and add the boiling water. Place pan over high heat and bring to a boil. Once boiling, reduce heat to medium-low, cover, and simmer for 12 minutes. Drain excess water.

2. Heat oil in a sauté pan over medium heat. Add garlic and onion and sauté for 2 minutes.

3. Add pepper and sauté for 4 minutes.

4. Add spinach and sauté until wilted, roughly 3–5 minutes. Remove pan from heat.

5. Add broth and stir to release the brown bits from the bottom of the pan.

6. Add the cooked couscous, lemon juice, and black pepper. Stir well to combine. Serve immediately.

PER SERVING | Calories: 141 | Fat: 1 g | Protein: 5 g | Sodium: 33 mg | Fiber: 2 g | Carbohydrates: 27 g | Sugar: 1 g

Apple Walnut Wheat Stuffing

Quick and easy to prepare using commercial salt-free bread, this stuffing adds interest to holiday or everyday meals. The nutty tang of the walnuts and wheat and subtle sweetness of the apples partners beautifully with roast chicken or turkey. Adapted from Gourmet Cooking without Salt.

INGREDIENTS | SERVES 8

1 tablespoon olive oil

3 cloves garlic, minced

1 large onion, chopped

3 medium tart green apples, diced

4 cups cubed salt-free wheat bread

¾ cup low-sodium chicken broth

½ cup chopped walnuts

1 tablespoon freshly squeezed lemon juice

1 tablespoon brown sugar

1½ teaspoons ground cinnamon

½ teaspoon freshly ground black pepper

¼ teaspoon ground nutmeg

1. Preheat oven to 325°F. Spray a lidded baking pan lightly with oil and set aside.

2. Heat the oil in a large sauté pan over medium. Add the garlic and onion and sauté for 2 minutes. Remove pan from heat.

3. Add the remaining ingredients and stir gently to combine.

4. Spread mixture in pan, cover, and place on middle rack in oven. Bake for 20 minutes.

5. Uncover and bake another 10 minutes. Remove from oven and serve immediately.

PER SERVING | Calories: 158 | Fat: 7 g | Protein: 3 g | Sodium: 13 mg | Fiber: 2 g | Carbohydrates: 22 g | Sugar: 9 g

Roasted Radishes and Brussels Sprouts

The roasting process mellows the flavor of both vegetables, leaving them ultra tender and caramelized. The pepper gains strength in the oven; use the lesser amount if you can't tolerate spice.

INGREDIENTS | SERVES 4

½ pound radishes

1 pound Brussels sprouts, halved

1 tablespoon freshly squeezed lemon juice

1½ teaspoons olive oil

¼–½ teaspoon freshly ground black pepper

Radish Facts

Radishes, like carrots, are root vegetables. Radishes and radish greens, as their edible leaves are known, have a pungent, peppery taste. This, along with their often vibrant colors, makes them a great choice for accenting salads. Roasting, braising, sautéing, or steaming radishes mellows their flavor significantly. Radishes are high in vitamin C and fiber and low in calories and sodium.

1. Preheat oven to 425°F. Spray a baking sheet lightly with oil and set aside.

2. Wash the radishes and pat dry. Halve or quarter depending upon size and place into a mixing bowl.

3. Add the halved Brussels sprouts, lemon juice, oil, and pepper and toss well to coat.

4. Arrange in a single layer on the baking sheet. Place on middle rack in oven and bake 25–30 minutes.

5. Remove from oven and serve immediately.

PER SERVING | Calories: 64 | Fat: 2 g | Protein: 3 g | Sodium: 45 mg | Fiber: 3 g | Carbohydrates: 10 g | Sugar: 3 g

Oven-Fried Green Tomatoes

If you like fried green tomatoes, you'll love this healthier version.
Soft and tender inside with a crisp outer coating, it's all of the flavor with none of the fat!

INGREDIENTS | SERVES 4

4 medium green tomatoes
1 egg white
½ cup salt-free bread crumbs
½ cup cornmeal
1 tablespoon grated Parmesan cheese
Freshly ground black pepper, to taste

1. Preheat oven to 425°F. Spray a baking sheet lightly with oil and set aside.

2. Wash and slice the tomatoes into thick, ½-inch rounds and set aside.

3. Place the egg white into a shallow bowl and beat.

4. Measure the bread crumbs and cornmeal into a second shallow bowl, add the Parmesan cheese and black pepper, and stir to combine.

5. Dip the tomato slices into the egg, then coat with bread crumbs. Place slices in a single layer on the baking sheet.

6. Place baking sheet on the middle rack in oven and bake for 15 minutes.

7. Gently flip the slices and return to the oven for another 10–15 minutes. Remove from oven and serve immediately.

PER SERVING | Calories: 148 | Fat: 1 g | Protein: 6 g | Sodium: 56 mg | Fiber: 3 g | Carbohydrates: 30 g | Sugar: 6 g

Carrots with Ginger, Cilantro, and Lime

Lively and flavorful, this carrot dish is a great partner for Indian fare or grilled meat. For more spice, add half a minced jalapeño pepper along with the other seasonings. Adapted from Fresh Magazine.

INGREDIENTS | SERVES 6

1 tablespoon minced fresh ginger

1½ teaspoons mustard seeds

1 teaspoon freshly ground black pepper

½ teaspoon ground coriander

½ teaspoon ground cumin

¼ teaspoon salt-free curry powder

2 pounds fresh carrots

¼ cup water

1 tablespoon canola oil

Juice of 1 fresh lime

¼ cup chopped fresh cilantro

What Are Mustard Seeds?

Mustard seeds are the spicy, edible seed of the mustard plant and come in three main types: white, brown, and black. White mustard seeds are the least pungent and are used to make standard yellow mustard, while the slightly spicier brown seeds are used to flavor Dijon mustard. Black seeds, the most pungent in taste, are often reserved for cooking. All mustard seeds contain cancer-fighting and anti-inflammatory compounds. Mustard seeds can be added to food and eaten either whole or ground.

1. Measure the ginger, mustard seeds, black pepper, coriander, cumin, and curry powder into a small bowl and set aside.

2. Peel the carrots and cut diagonally into roughly ½-inch slices.

3. Place a sauté pan over medium heat. Add the water, oil, and carrots to the pan and bring to a boil. Cover pan and cook, shaking occasionally, until carrots are just barely tender, about 7 minutes.

4. Uncover the pan and continue to cook until carrots begin to sizzle in the oil, about 2 minutes.

5. Add the spice mixture and cook, stirring constantly, for 2 minutes. Remove from heat.

6. Add the lime juice and cilantro and stir to combine. Serve immediately.

PER SERVING | Calories: 74 | Fat: 2 g | Protein: 1 g | Sodium: 117 mg | Fiber: 4 g | Carbohydrates: 12 g | Sugar: 7 g

Baked Spinach and Pea Risotto

There's something magical about the combination of tastes and textures in this risotto. The wine, broth, and cheese lend so much flavor, and the creaminess keeps you coming back for more. For those concerned about the sodium in the cheese, eliminate it altogether. Adapted from Real Simple.

INGREDIENTS | SERVES 6

1 tablespoon unsalted butter
1 shallot, chopped
Freshly ground black pepper, to taste
½ cup dry white wine
3 cups low-sodium chicken broth
1 cup arborio rice
1 cup frozen peas
2 cups chopped fresh baby spinach
¼ cup grated Parmesan cheese

Sodium in Frozen Vegetables

Many frozen vegetables are just that, frozen vegetables. But others contain things you don't want, like added salt and sauces. Even "plain" veggies may have been treated in such a way that elevates their sodium content. When selecting frozen vegetables, check nutrition facts carefully to ensure you're buying the vegetables you want, without anything else.

1. Preheat oven to 425°F.

2. Place a Dutch oven or similar lidded casserole pan over medium-high heat. Add the butter. Once melted, add the shallot and black pepper and sauté for 3 minutes.

3. Add the wine and cook, stirring, until almost evaporated, 2–3 minutes.

4. Add the broth and rice and bring to a boil.

5. Once boiling, cover the pot and transfer to the middle rack in the oven. Bake for 20 minutes, until rice is tender and creamy.

6. Remove from oven. Add the peas, spinach, and Parmesan and stir well to combine. Season with additional ground black pepper, to taste, if desired. Serve immediately.

PER SERVING | Calories: 209 | Fat: 4 g | Protein: 7 g | Sodium: 110 mg | Fiber: 1 g | Carbohydrates: 32 g | Sugar: 2 g

Curried Butternut Squash

A dish to turn to for both casual meals and holiday affairs. The roasting process brings out the sweetness of the squash, and the curry adds a savory dimension that's truly out of this world. Adapted from Taste of Home Dinner on a Dime.

INGREDIENTS | SERVES 6

1 medium butternut squash
2 tablespoons unsalted butter
1 teaspoon salt-free curry powder

1. Preheat oven to 450°F. Get out a 9" × 13" baking dish and set aside.

2. Place squash on a cutting board. Trim off the top and bottom, then carefully peel. Slice in half and remove seeds using a spoon. Cut into 1-inch cubes and set aside.

3. Place butter in baking dish and put pan into the oven. Watch, and remove as soon as the butter has melted. Sprinkle curry powder over the melted butter, then add the cubed squash and toss until evenly coated.

4. Place baking pan on middle rack in oven and roast 20–25 minutes, until squash is tender and very lightly browned. Remove from oven and serve immediately.

PER SERVING | Calories: 75 | Fat: 4 g | Protein: 1 g | Sodium: 5 mg | Fiber: 1 g | Carbohydrates: 11 g | Sugar: 2 g

Whipped Sweet Potatoes

*Perfect for holiday meals, this light and creamy concoction
of sweet potato has hints of orange and vanilla.*

INGREDIENTS | SERVES 6

3 medium–large sweet potatoes

3 tablespoons unsalted butter

3 tablespoons brown sugar

1 tablespoon freshly squeezed orange juice

¼ teaspoon pure vanilla extract

Whipped Butternut Squash

Puréed winter squash is a favorite recipe in New England and is super easy to make. Peel a medium butternut squash, seed, then cut into chunks. Place chunks in a microwave-safe bowl, add ¼ cup water, and cover with plastic wrap. Microwave on high for 10 minutes. Transfer contents to a food processor, add a tablespoon of low-sodium chicken or vegetable broth, and purée. Season to taste.

1. Peel sweet potatoes and cut into chunks. Place chunks in a pot and add enough water to cover by 1 or 2 inches. Place pot over high heat and bring to a boil. Once boiling, lower heat slightly and continue cooking until tender, about 20 minutes.

2. Drain pot. Place ⅓ of the sweet potatoes into a food processor, add 1 tablespoon butter, and purée. Remove to a bowl. Repeat process with remaining sweet potatoes and butter.

3. Add the brown sugar, orange juice, and vanilla to the bowl of whipped sweet potatoes and stir well to combine. Serve immediately.

PER SERVING | Calories: 136 | Fat: 5 g | Protein: 1 g | Sodium: 23 mg | Fiber: 2 g | Carbohydrates: 20 g | Sugar: 11 g

Red Potatoes with Peas, Parsley, and Mustard

Mustard, wine, and shallot meld together to elevate simple peas and potatoes to new heights. Excellent served hot or cold. Add chopped hard-boiled egg for extra protein. Adapted from the American Medical Association Family Health Cookbook.

INGREDIENTS | SERVES 4

1½ pounds red potatoes

1 cup fresh or frozen peas

¼ cup dry white wine

1 shallot, chopped

2 tablespoons salt-free prepared mustard

1 tablespoon olive oil

Freshly ground black pepper, to taste

¼ cup chopped fresh parsley

1. Scrub the potatoes and cut into 1½-inch chunks.

2. Bring a large pot of water to boil, add the potatoes, and cook until tender, roughly 10–15 minutes.

3. If using fresh peas, add them to the boiling water during the last 5 minutes of cooking; if using frozen peas, add 2 minutes before the end.

4. Drain the potatoes and peas into a colander and set aside. Do not wash the pot.

5. Return the pot to the stove, place over high heat, and add the wine and shallots. Cook for 1–2 minutes to soften, then remove the pot from the heat and whisk in the mustard, oil, and black pepper.

6. Add the potatoes and peas back into the pot and toss well to coat. Add the parsley and stir. Serve immediately.

PER SERVING | Calories: 215 | Fat: 3 g | Protein: 4 g | Sodium: 10 mg | Fiber: 4 g | Carbohydrates: 39 g | Sugar: 3 g

Wheat Berry Pilaf with Roasted Vegetables

Chewy, bright, and incredibly flavorful, thanks to the quartet of roasted veggies.
This makes a great potluck dish and may be served either hot or cold.

INGREDIENTS | SERVES 6

¾ cup parboiled dry wheat berries (e.g., Nature's Earthly Choice)

2 cups water

1 small bulb fennel

3 medium carrots, sliced

1 medium red onion, diced

8 cloves garlic, roughly chopped

1 teaspoon olive oil

¼–½ teaspoon ground cinnamon, to taste

Freshly ground black pepper, to taste

What Are Wheat Berries?

Wheat berries are individual kernels of wheat with the outer husk removed. They are a whole grain, containing all the beneficial parts of the plant. Wheat berries come in red and white varieties, can be cooked and eaten whole, or ground into flour. They're high in fiber and protein, low in fat, and sodium free. When cooked, they have a chewy texture and a pleasant, slightly nutty flavor. Standard wheat berries take about an hour to cook; look for parboiled (partly cooked) dry wheat berries to speed preparation. Nature's Earthly Choice is an excellent brand and is sold in many supermarkets and natural food stores.

1. Preheat oven to 425°F. Lightly spray a baking sheet with oil and set aside.

2. Place wheat berries and water in a saucepan and bring to a boil over high heat. Once boiling, reduce heat to low, cover, and simmer for 15 minutes. Drain any excess water. Set aside.

3. Wash and dry the fennel. Dice the white bulb and stems and place into a mixing bowl. Coarsely chop the green fronds and set aside.

4. Add the carrots, onion, and garlic to the bowl of fennel. Add a teaspoon of olive oil and toss well to coat.

5. Arrange veggies in a single layer on the prepared baking sheet. Place on middle rack in oven and roast for 15 minutes. Remove from oven.

6. Place in a bowl, along with the cooked wheat berries, chopped fennel fronds, cinnamon, and freshly ground black pepper to taste. Stir well to combine.

7. Serve immediately or cover and refrigerate until serving.

PER SERVING | Calories: 211 | Fat: 2 g | Protein: 7 g | Sodium: 79 mg | Fiber: 9 g | Carbohydrates: 43 g | Sugar: 3 g

Whole-Wheat Couscous with Plums, Ginger, and Allspice

An appealing complexity of flavors in a super simple package.
Light, fragrant, and incredibly healthy, this side dish is terrific served warm or cold.

INGREDIENTS | SERVES 6

1½ cups water

1 cup whole-wheat couscous

2 ripe plums, diced

3 scallions, sliced

2 teaspoons minced fresh ginger

¼ cup chopped walnuts

¼ teaspoon freshly ground black pepper

¼ teaspoon ground allspice

1. Measure water into a saucepan and bring to a boil over high heat. Once boiling, stir in the couscous, reduce heat to medium-low, cover, and simmer for 2 minutes.

2. Remove pot from heat, remove lid, and fluff couscous with a fork. Let stand for 5 minutes.

3. Place remaining ingredients into a mixing bowl. Add couscous and toss well to combine.

4. Serve immediately or cover and refrigerate until serving.

PER SERVING | Calories: 138 | Fat: 4 g | Protein: 4 g | Sodium: 0 mg | Fiber: 2 g | Carbohydrates: 22 g | Sugar: 3 g

Hearty Cabbage and Noodles

Healthy, tasty, and flavorful, this salt-free side also makes a great vegetarian main course.
Adapted from the American Heart Association's Low-Salt Cookbook.

INGREDIENTS | SERVES 6

8 ounces yolkless wide egg noodles

1 tablespoon olive oil

½ medium head green cabbage, chopped

1 medium onion, chopped

1 teaspoon caraway seeds

Freshly ground black pepper, to taste

1. Prepare noodles according to package directions, omitting salt. Drain and set aside.

2. Heat oil in a large sauté pan over medium heat. Add cabbage and onion and sauté for 5–8 minutes, until tender crisp.

3. Stir in noodles, caraway seeds, and freshly ground black pepper, to taste.

4. Serve immediately.

PER SERVING | Calories: 138 | Fat: 3 g | Protein: 4 g | Sodium: 22 mg | Fiber: 3 g | Carbohydrates: 23 g | Sugar: 3 g

Garlic Rosemary Mashed Potatoes

Potatoes often fall flat without the boost of salt, but these salt-free mashed potatoes, made without butter and milk, too, may be the best you've ever had.

INGREDIENTS | SERVES 6

6 cups cubed red potatoes

6 cloves garlic

2 tablespoons olive oil

¼ cup low-sodium vegetable broth

1 teaspoon unflavored rice wine vinegar

1 teaspoon ground rosemary

½ teaspoon ground white pepper

¼ teaspoon ground dry mustard

Rosemary Facts

Rosemary is a perennial herb with a strong taste and fragrance. It grows in sturdy sprigs with leaves reminiscent of soft pine needles. Rosemary can be used either fresh or dried, and is often ground into a fragrant powder for ease in use. It contains iron and several antioxidants believed to ward against neurological disorders such as Alzheimer's and Parkinson's disease.

1. Place potatoes in a pot and add enough water to cover. Place pot over high heat and bring to a boil. Once boiling, reduce heat to medium-high and simmer for 15 minutes.

2. Measure remaining ingredients into a food processor and purée until smooth.

3. Remove pot from heat and drain. Mash potatoes. Add dressing and stir well to combine.

4. Serve immediately.

PER SERVING | Calories: 181 | Fat: 4 g | Protein: 3 g | Sodium: 13 mg | Fiber: 3 g | Carbohydrates: 32 g | Sugar: 1 g

Southwestern Rice Pilaf

Filling and flavorful, this easy rice pilaf partners perfectly with Tex-Mex dishes, burgers, and refried beans. Adapted from Fine Cooking.

INGREDIENTS | SERVES 4

1 tablespoon olive oil

1 medium red onion, diced

4 cloves garlic, minced

1 medium red bell pepper, diced

1 small green bell pepper, diced

2 teaspoons salt-free chili seasoning

1 teaspoon ground cumin

1½ cups long-grain rice

2½ cups low-sodium vegetable broth

1 (15-ounce) can no-salt-added diced tomatoes

1 jalapeño pepper, minced

¼ cup chopped fresh cilantro

1. Heat oil in a large lidded saucepan over medium heat. Add the onion, garlic, and bell peppers and sauté for 2 minutes.

2. Add the chili powder and cumin and sauté for 3 minutes.

3. Add the rice and stir well to coat. Reduce heat to medium-low and cook, stirring, for 2 minutes.

4. Add the broth and tomatoes and stir well. Raise heat to high and bring to a boil. Once boiling, reduce heat to low, cover securely, and simmer for 18 minutes. Remove from heat and let sit for 5 minutes.

5. Remove lid, add the jalapeño and cilantro, and gently fold in. Serve immediately.

PER SERVING | Calories: 304 | Fat: 4 g | Protein: 7 g | Sodium: 105 mg | Fiber: 4 g | Carbohydrates: 57 g | Sugar: 5 g

Garlic Steamed Squash

*One of the simplest sides ever. Slice yellow squash and zucchini,
toss them into a steamer with some garlic cloves, and in 10 minutes it's ready!*

INGREDIENTS | SERVES 4

2 small–medium yellow squash
2 small–medium zucchini
6 cloves garlic, peeled
Ground white pepper, to taste

Garlic Facts

Sometimes referred to as the stinking rose, garlic has been used since ancient times as both food and medicine. It can be eaten raw, cooked, dried, and ground, and is used to flavor cuisines from around the world. Garlic contains manganese, vitamins B_6 and C, and several phytochemicals believed to fight disease.

1. Trim the squash and zucchini and cut into 1-inch rounds.

2. Fill a steamer pot about 1 inch deep with water. Place pot over high heat and bring to a boil.

3. Place the veggies and garlic into the steamer basket. Place the steamer basket into the pot and cover tightly with lid. Steam for 10 minutes.

4. Remove pot from heat and carefully remove lid. Pluck garlic cloves from pot and gently mash with a fork.

5. Transfer the steamed veggies to a serving bowl, add the garlic and white pepper, and toss gently to coat. Serve immediately.

PER SERVING | Calories: 38 | Fat: 0 g | Protein: 2 g | Sodium: 5 mg | Fiber: 2 g | Carbohydrates: 8 g | Sugar: 4 g

Peppery Swiss Chard

Swiss chard has a flavor akin to spinach, with vibrantly colorful celery-like stalks. This makes an interesting and highly nutritious side, perfect for those who enjoy their spice. If you're someone who doesn't, simply reduce or omit the pepper flakes.

INGREDIENTS | SERVES 4

1 bunch fresh Swiss chard

2 teaspoons olive oil

2 cloves garlic, slivered finely

¼ teaspoon dried red pepper flakes

Freshly ground black pepper, to taste

Swiss Chard Facts

Swiss chard is a dark, leafy green with colorful stalks akin to celery. It has a somewhat bitter taste that mellows with cooking, and is particularly well suited to sautéing with a little olive oil and garlic. Swiss chard is an excellent source of vitamins A, C, and K, manganese, potassium, iron, and fiber, and contains antioxidants linked to the prevention of cancer and cardiovascular disease.

1. Wash the Swiss chard well, then pat dry. Trim each piece by removing most of the stalk, leaving just 1 or 2 inches of stalk beneath each leafy portion. Chop the leaves and stems into 2-inch pieces and set aside.

2. Heat oil in a sauté pan over medium heat. Add the garlic and sauté for 1 minute.

3. Add Swiss chard and sauté for 8 minutes.

4. Remove from heat and stir in the red pepper flakes. Season to taste with freshly ground black pepper. Serve immediately.

PER SERVING | Calories: 29 | Fat: 2 g | Protein: 0 g | Sodium: 76 mg | Fiber: 1 g | Carbohydrates: 2 g | Sugar: 0 g

Sundried Tomato Couscous with Pine Nuts, Garlic, and Basil

*Sundried tomatoes do double duty in this flavorful whole-grain couscous,
providing an astronomical amount of flavor with absolutely no salt.
Select sundried tomatoes stored without oil.*

INGREDIENTS | SERVES 4

1 cup chopped sundried tomatoes
2 cups boiling water
1 cup dry whole-grain couscous
2 teaspoons olive oil
4 cloves garlic, minced
⅓ cup pine nuts
¼ teaspoon freshly ground black pepper
2 tablespoons chopped fresh basil

1. Place the sundried tomatoes in a small bowl and add the boiling water. Let sit for 15 minutes.

2. Pour the soaking liquid into a measuring cup and add enough water to make 2 cups. Set tomatoes aside.

3. Pour liquid into a saucepan and bring to a boil over high heat. Once boiling, stir in the couscous, reduce heat to medium-low, cover, and simmer for 2 minutes.

4. Remove pot from heat, remove lid, and fluff couscous with a fork. Set aside to cool for 5 minutes.

5. Heat olive oil in a sauté pan over medium heat. Add the tomatoes, garlic, and pine nuts and sauté for 3 minutes. Remove from heat.

6. Add couscous, pepper, and basil and toss well to combine. Serve immediately.

PER SERVING | Calories: 275 | Fat: 11 g | Protein: 8 g | Sodium: 282 mg | Fiber: 4 g | Carbohydrates: 37 g | Sugar: 6 g

CHAPTER 16

Cookies, Brownies, and Bars

Peanut Butter Chocolate Chip Blondies

The stellar combination of peanut butter and chocolate in a moist cookie bar.
For a yummy vegan version, substitute egg replacement powder for the egg whites.

INGREDIENTS | YIELDS 2 DOZEN

¼ cup salt-free peanut butter
¾ cup light brown sugar
½ cup unsweetened applesauce
¼ cup canola oil
2 egg whites
1 tablespoon pure vanilla extract
2 teaspoons sodium-free baking powder
1 cup unbleached all-purpose flour
½ cup white whole-wheat flour
½ cup semisweet chocolate chips

1. Preheat oven to 350°F. Grease and flour a 9" × 13" baking pan and set aside.

2. Measure the peanut butter, sugar, applesauce, oil, egg whites, and vanilla into a mixing bowl and stir well to combine.

3. Add the baking powder and mix.

4. Gradually add in the flours, stirring well.

5. Fold in the chocolate chips.

6. Spread batter in prepared pan and smooth to even. Place pan on middle rack in oven and bake for 30 minutes. Remove from oven and place on wire rack to cool.

7. Cool before cutting into bars and serving.

PER SERVING | Calories: 18 | Fat: 5 g | Protein: 2 g |
Sodium: 7 mg | Fiber: 1 g | Carbohydrates: 17 g | Sugar: 10 g

Vegan Chocolate Chip Cookies

Subtly sweet and absolutely delicious, these cookies have a dry crumb that's downright addictive. Partner with nondairy milk for the full cookie experience. Adapted from Leslie Cerier, the Organic Gourmet.

INGREDIENTS | YIELDS 3 DOZEN

1¼ cups unbleached all-purpose flour
¾ cup whole-wheat flour
⅓ cup canola oil
⅓ cup pure maple syrup
1 tablespoon pure vanilla extract
¾ cup semisweet chocolate chips
2 tablespoons water

Is Chocolate Vegan?

Happily, yes. Although some brands of chocolate contain milk derivatives, others do not. When in doubt, check product packaging carefully. Trader Joe's and Whole Foods sell store-brand chocolate chips that are 100 percent vegan and tasty. Many health food stores and supermarkets also stock vegan-friendly chocolate morsels and bars. If you can't find them locally, shop online.

1. Preheat oven to 375°F. Take out 2 baking sheets and set aside.

2. Place the flours, oil, maple syrup, and vanilla into a large mixing bowl and stir to combine. The mixture will be quite dry and crumbly.

3. Add the chocolate chips and stir well.

4. Add the water and stir to incorporate.

5. Scoop the dough ½ tablespoon at a time and shape into cookies. Place cookies on the baking sheets and bake on middle rack in oven for 10 minutes.

6. Remove from oven and transfer to a wire rack to cool. Store cookies in an airtight container.

PER SERVING | Calories: 74 | Fat: 3 g | Protein: 1 g | Sodium: 1 mg | Fiber: 0 g | Carbohydrates: 10 g | Sugar: 4 g

Vegan Orange Cranberry Cookies

A citrus twist on vegan chocolate chip cookies, these have a bright orange flavor and burst of sweetness from the dried cranberries.

INGREDIENTS | YIELDS 3 DOZEN

2 cups white whole-wheat flour

⅓ cup canola oil

⅓ cup pure maple syrup

2 tablespoons freshly squeezed orange juice

Grated zest of 1 fresh orange

¾ cup dried cranberries

1. Preheat oven to 375°F. Take out 2 baking sheets and set aside.

2. Place the flour, oil, maple syrup, orange juice, and zest into a large mixing bowl and stir to combine. The mixture will be quite dry and crumbly.

3. Add the cranberries and stir well.

4. Scoop the dough ½ tablespoon at a time and shape into cookies. Place cookies on the baking sheets and bake on middle rack in oven for 10 minutes.

5. Remove from oven and transfer to a wire rack to cool. Store cookies in an airtight container.

PER SERVING (PER COOKIE) | Calories: 56 | Fat: 2 g | Protein: 1 g | Sodium: 1 mg | Fiber: 1 g | Carbohydrates: 9 g | Sugar: 3 g

Vegan Lemon Drops

Like the candy, but better! These vegan cookies pack a huge pucker punch, softened by the sweetness of white chocolate chips. For another great taste, swap the lemon juice and zest for lime.

INGREDIENTS | YIELDS 3 DOZEN

1¼ cups unbleached all-purpose flour

¾ cup white whole-wheat flour

⅓ cup canola oil

⅓ cup pure maple syrup

Juice and grated zest of 1 fresh lemon

¾ cup vegan white chocolate chips

Vegan White Chocolate

Vegan white chocolate chips are sold at some supermarkets, natural food stores, and online. Although they may be more difficult to find, they're worth the effort. In addition to their sweet, creamy taste, some white vegan chips, such as Oppenheimer, aren't just low in sodium, they're sodium free!

1. Preheat oven to 375°F. Take out 2 baking sheets and set aside.

2. Place the flours, oil, maple syrup, lemon juice, and zest into a large mixing bowl and stir to combine. The mixture will be quite dry and crumbly.

3. Add the white chocolate chips and stir well.

4. Scoop the dough ½ tablespoon at a time and shape into cookies. Place cookies on the baking sheets and bake on middle rack in oven for 10 minutes.

5. Remove from oven and transfer to a wire rack to cool. Store cookies in an airtight container.

PER SERVING (PER COOKIE) | Calories: 73 | Fat: 3 g | Protein: 1 g | Sodium: 1 mg | Fiber: 0 g | Carbohydrates: 10 g | Sugar: 4 g

Chocolate Pomegranate Brownies

Moist with an undeniably decadent taste, every bite of these brownies is infused with the dark sweetness of pomegranate juice. These make a spectacular treat for special occasions.

INGREDIENTS | YIELDS 16

¾ cup unsweetened cocoa powder
¾ cup unbleached all-purpose flour
¾ cup sugar
1 cup pomegranate juice (e.g., Pom)
2 eggs
½ cup canola oil
1 teaspoon sodium-free baking powder

1. Preheat oven to 350°F. Grease and flour an 8-inch square pan and set aside.

2. Place ingredients into a mixing bowl and beat for 2 minutes.

3. Pour batter into prepared pan. Place pan on middle rack in oven and bake for 30 minutes.

4. Remove from oven and place on wire rack to cool. Cool to touch before cutting into squares and serving.

PER SERVING (PER BROWNIE) | Calories: 144 | Fat: 8 g | Protein: 2 g | Sodium: 11 mg | Fiber: 1 g | Carbohydrates: 18 g | Sugar: 11 g

Ginger Snaps

Fans of classic ginger snaps will love these dark, aromatic cookies with a crisp bite. And they're not just low in sodium, they're low in fat, too!

INGREDIENTS | YIELDS 18

4 tablespoons unsalted butter
½ cup light brown sugar
2 tablespoons molasses
1 egg white
2½ teaspoons ground ginger
¼ teaspoon ground allspice
1 teaspoon sodium-free baking soda
½ cup unbleached all-purpose flour
½ cup white whole-wheat flour
1 tablespoon demerara sugar

Cookie Baking Tip

Never place cookie dough onto a hot baking sheet; cookies will precook before reaching the oven and end up overly dark. For perfect results, use multiple baking sheets. Measure dough onto a cool baking sheet, bake, then remove cookies to a wire rack. Set the hot baking sheet aside to cool, and start afresh with a second baking sheet.

1. Preheat oven to 375°F. Line a baking sheet with parchment and set aside.

2. Place the butter, sugar, and molasses into a mixing bowl and beat well to combine.

3. Add the egg white, ginger, and allspice and mix well.

4. Stir in the baking soda, then gradually add the flours. Beat until combined, scraping down the sides of the bowl as necessary.

5. Scoop the dough by tablespoonfuls and roll into small balls. Place balls on lined baking sheet and press down using a glass dipped in the demerara sugar.

6. Place baking sheet on middle rack in oven and bake for 10 minutes.

7. Remove from oven and transfer cookies to a wire rack to cool. Store in an airtight container.

PER SERVING | Calories: 81 | Fat: 2 g | Protein: 1 g | Sodium: 6 mg | Fiber: 0 g | Carbohydrates: 14 g | Sugar: 8 g

Carrot Cake Cookies

Soft whole-grain cookies with the taste and texture of carrot cake! To make the oat flour, measure rolled oats into a food processor and pulse until fine.

INGREDIENTS | YIELDS 3 DOZEN

3 medium carrots, shredded
1½ cups unbleached all-purpose flour
¾ cup oat flour
¾ cup light brown sugar
1 egg white
⅓ cup canola oil
1 tablespoon pure vanilla extract
1 teaspoon sodium-free baking powder
1½ teaspoons ground cinnamon
½ teaspoon ground nutmeg
¼ teaspoon ground ginger
⅛ teaspoon ground cloves

1. Preheat oven to 375°F. Line a baking sheet with parchment and set aside.

2. Place all the ingredients into a mixing bowl and stir well to combine. Dough will be quite sticky.

3. Drop by tablespoonfuls onto lined baking sheet. Place sheet on middle rack in oven and bake for 12 minutes.

4. Remove from oven and transfer cookies to a wire rack to cool. Store in an airtight container.

PER SERVING (PER COOKIE) | Calories: 67 | Fat: 2 g | Protein: 1 g | Sodium: 7 mg | Fiber: 0 g | Carbohydrates: 10 g | Sugar: 4 g

Ice Cream Scoops Make Perfect Cookies!

Instead of fumbling with table spoons, scoop out cookie dough using a small retractable ice cream scoop. Ice cream scoops produce uniform, picture-perfect cookies and reduce hassle and mess. Small scoops are sold at kitchenware shops and other stores as well as online.

Chai Oatmeal Cookies

Scented with a quintet of spices, these cookies are best served with an ice cold glass of milk or nondairy milk. Add chocolate chips, dried fruit, or chopped nuts if desired.

INGREDIENTS | YIELDS 2 DOZEN

1½ cups old-fashioned rolled oats

½ cup unbleached all-purpose flour

½ cup light brown sugar

¼ cup sugar

⅓ cup unsalted butter, softened

1 egg white

1 tablespoon pure vanilla extract

1 teaspoon sodium-free baking powder

1½ teaspoons ground cinnamon

¾ teaspoon ground cardamom

½ teaspoon ground ginger

¼ teaspoon ground allspice

¼ teaspoon ground cloves

1. Preheat oven to 375°F. Line a baking sheet with parchment and set aside.

2. Measure oats, flour, sugars, and butter into a mixing bowl and beat well.

3. Add remaining ingredients and stir to combine.

4. Drop batter by tablespoonfuls onto the lined baking sheet. Place sheet on middle rack in oven and bake for 10 minutes.

5. Remove from oven and transfer to wire rack to cool. Store in an airtight container.

PER SERVING (PER COOKIE) | Calories: 78 | Fat: 3 g | Protein: 1 g | Sodium: 4 mg | Fiber: 0 g | Carbohydrates: 12 g | Sugar: 6 g

Lemon Poppy Seed Cookies

Soft, chewy cookies with the bright zing of citrus and contrasting bite of poppy seeds.

INGREDIENTS | YIELDS 2 DOZEN

5 tablespoons unsalted butter, softened
¾ cup sugar
1 egg white
Juice and grated zest of 1 fresh lemon
1 teaspoon pure vanilla extract
1 teaspoon sodium-free baking powder
1½ teaspoons poppy seeds
1½ cups unbleached all-purpose flour

What Are Poppy Seeds?

Poppy seeds are the tiny seeds of the opium poppy, the same plant that produces the opiate drug. Although the small amount of poppy seeds used in standard recipes won't produce a sensory effect, it could trigger a false positive in a urine drug test for up to two days following ingestion.

1. Preheat oven to 375°F. Line a baking sheet with parchment and set aside.

2. Measure butter and sugar into a mixing bowl and beat until fluffy.

3. Add remaining ingredients and stir until combined.

4. Scoop batter by tablespoonfuls onto lined baking sheet.

5. Place baking sheet on middle rack in oven and bake for 8 minutes. Remove from oven and transfer to a wire rack to cool. Store in an airtight container.

PER SERVING (PER COOKIE) | Calories: 75 | Fat: 2 g | Protein: 1 g | Sodium: 3 mg | Fiber: 0 g | Carbohydrates: 12 g | Sugar: 6 g

Coconut Chocolate Chip Blondies

Irresistibly delicious cookie bars. Use dark, semisweet, or milk chocolate chips and add chopped almonds to the batter too if desired.

INGREDIENTS | YIELDS 16

5 tablespoons unsalted butter, softened
⅔ cup light brown sugar
2 egg whites
2 teaspoons pure vanilla extract
½ teaspoon sodium-free baking powder
¾ cup white whole-wheat flour
½ cup unbleached all-purpose flour
¼ cup unsweetened shredded coconut
½ cup chocolate chips

1. Preheat oven to 350°F. Grease and flour an 8-inch baking pan and set aside.

2. Place the butter and brown sugar into a mixing bowl and beat well to combine.

3. Stir in the egg whites and vanilla.

4. Add the baking powder and mix.

5. Gradually add in the flours and coconut, then fold in the chocolate chips.

6. Transfer batter to the prepared pan and smooth to even. Place on middle rack in oven and bake for 30 minutes.

7. Remove from oven and place pan on wire rack to cool. Cool to touch before cutting into squares and serving.

PER SERVING (PER BLONDIE) | Calories: 150 | Fat: 7 g | Protein: 2 g | Sodium: 11 mg | Fiber: 1 g | Carbohydrates: 21 g | Sugar: 13 g

Banana Bars

Soft, moist, and satisfying, these cake-like bars are packed with bright banana flavor. Egg replacement powder is sold at many supermarkets, health food stores, and online; ground flaxseed or an egg white may be substituted instead.

INGREDIENTS | YIELDS 16

Egg replacement powder for 1 egg
2 ripe medium bananas, mashed
½ cup light brown sugar
4 tablespoons canola oil
2 teaspoons pure vanilla extract
1 tablespoon sodium-free baking powder
½ teaspoon ground cardamom
⅛ teaspoon ground cinnamon
¾ cup white whole-wheat flour
⅓ cup unbleached all-purpose flour

Cookie Baking Tip

When baking cookie bars, allow them to cool fully in the pan before slicing and removing. This keeps the edges intact and helps ensure your cookie bars look picture perfect. To get evenly sized bars, slice halfway through the pan, then divide each half in half, and slice again.

1. Preheat oven to 375°F. Grease and flour an 8-inch square baking pan and set aside.

2. Prepare the egg replacement powder according to package directions and pour into a mixing bowl.

3. Add the mashed banana, brown sugar, oil, vanilla, baking powder, cardamom, and cinnamon and stir well to combine.

4. Add the flours and stir well. The batter will be quite sticky.

5. Pour into prepared pan and smooth to even. Place pan on middle rack in oven and bake for 25 minutes.

6. Remove from oven and place on a wire rack to cool. Slice into squares. Store in an airtight container until serving.

PER SERVING | Calories: 107 | Fat: 4 g | Protein: 2 g | Sodium: 15 mg | Fiber: 1 g | Carbohydrates: 16 g | Sugar: 9 g

CHAPTER 17

Desserts

Apple, Pear, and Cranberry Crisp with Fresh Ginger

Juicy fruit under a sweet whole-grain crust. What's not to love? This fabulous crisp is a perfect vehicle for fall fruit. Vary the types of apples and pears to subtly change the flavor, or swap them altogether for a different fruit or fruits.

INGREDIENTS | SERVES 8

3 medium apples

3 medium pears

1 cup fresh or frozen cranberries

1 tablespoon freshly squeezed lemon juice

2 tablespoons minced fresh ginger

⅓ cup sugar

1 cup rolled oats

⅓ cup white whole-wheat flour

½ cup light brown sugar

1 teaspoon pure vanilla extract

1 teaspoon ground cinnamon

¼ teaspoon ground allspice

⅛ teaspoon ground cardamom

3 tablespoons unsalted butter

Freezer Alert

Fresh cranberries are often on sale around the holidays. Buy an extra bag or two and pop them into the freezer for future use. If kept frozen, cranberries will last for months and can be added to many recipes, often without defrosting.

1. Preheat oven to 400°F. Take out a 2-quart baking pan and set aside.

2. Peel and core the apples and pears, and slice each into 16 wedges.

3. Place into a mixing bowl, add the cranberries, lemon juice, ginger, and sugar and toss well to coat.

4. Turn mixture out into the baking pan and set aside.

5. Place the oats, flour, sugar, vanilla, and spices into a mixing bowl and stir to combine.

6. Cut the butter into the mixture using your (freshly washed) hands and process until a wet crumb has formed. Sprinkle mixture over fruit.

7. Place on middle rack in oven and bake for 30 minutes. Remove from oven and place on a wire rack to cool.

PER SERVING | Calories: 263 | Fat: 5 g | Protein: 2 g | Sodium: 6 mg | Fiber: 6 g | Carbohydrates: 55 g | Sugar: 36 g

Mini Cornmeal Rhubarb Crisps

Soft lemon-flavored fruit blanketed beneath a crunchy, sweet cornmeal crust. These little crisps make a sensational spring dessert for company.

INGREDIENTS | SERVES 4

3 cups sliced fresh rhubarb

3 tablespoons sugar

2 tablespoons freshly squeezed lemon juice

Grated zest of 1 fresh lemon

¼ cup cornmeal

3 tablespoons light brown sugar

2 tablespoons old-fashioned rolled oats

2 tablespoons nonhydrogenated vegetable shortening

Rhubarb Facts

Rhubarb is an easy-to-grow perennial vegetable with poisonous green leaves and edible pink or red stalks. Rhubarb has a very tart flavor, which is counteracted by the addition of sugar, so it's seen most often in baked goods and desserts. Rhubarb's high acidity may cause a reaction with some metal cookware, so cook or bake rhubarb in stainless steel or nonstick pans whenever possible.

1. Preheat oven to 375°F. Take out 4 (roughly 4-inch) ramekins.

2. Place the rhubarb, sugar, and lemon juice into a mixing bowl and toss well to coat. Divide mixture evenly between the ramekins.

3. Place the lemon zest, cornmeal, brown sugar, and oats into another mixing bowl and whisk well to combine.

4. Add the shortening to the bowl and work into the mixture using your (freshly washed) hands. When a sturdy crumb has been achieved, sprinkle mixture over the rhubarb, dividing evenly.

5. Place ramekins on the middle rack in the oven and bake for 20 minutes.

6. Remove from oven. Set aside to cool for a few minutes. Serve warm.

PER SERVING | Calories: 189 | Fat: 7 g | Protein: 2 g | Sodium: 10 mg | Fiber: 2 g | Carbohydrates: 32 g | Sugar: 20 g

Mango Crumble

Sink your teeth into tender chunks of mango with a cinnamon-scented crust.
For a juicier filling, omit the cornstarch.

INGREDIENTS | SERVES 8

2 barely ripe mangoes
2 tablespoons light brown sugar
1 tablespoon cornstarch
1½ teaspoons minced fresh ginger
½ cup unbleached all-purpose flour
½ cup white whole-wheat flour
½ cup sugar
1 teaspoon ground cinnamon
¼ teaspoon ground ginger
3 tablespoons unsalted butter

1. Preheat oven to 350°F. Take out an 8-inch square baking pan and set aside.

2. Peel mangoes and cut into 1-inch chunks. Place in a mixing bowl.

3. Add the brown sugar, cornstarch, and minced ginger and toss to coat. Turn mixture out onto the baking pan and spread to even.

4. In another bowl, whisk together the flours, sugar, cinnamon, and ginger.

5. Cut the butter into small pieces and add to the bowl. Work butter into the mixture using your (freshly washed) hands until it resembles damp sand and sticks together when squeezed. Sprinkle mixture evenly over the fruit.

6. Place pan on middle rack in oven and bake for 25–30 minutes, until tender. Remove from oven and place on wire rack to cool. Serve warm or cool.

PER SERVING | Calories: 190 | Fat: 5 g | Protein: 3 g | Sodium: 3 mg | Fiber: 2 g | Carbohydrates: 37 g | Sugar: 23 g

Fruit Pizza

A sweetly stunning showcase for your favorite fresh fruit. Mascarpone cheese is sold in the specialty cheese section of many supermarkets.

INGREDIENTS | SERVES 12

4 tablespoons unsalted butter

¾ cup sugar

1 teaspoon pure vanilla extract

Juice and grated zest of 1 fresh lemon

1⅔ cups unbleached all-purpose flour

4 tablespoons low-fat milk

½ cup mascarpone cheese

2 tablespoons nonfat sour cream

⅔ cup powdered sugar

3 cups sliced assorted fresh fruit

Mascarpone Cheese

Mascarpone (pronounced mas-kahr-POH-nay) is a light, sweet, and creamy Italian cheese. Delicious in desserts, spread thinly on toast, or swirled into hot pasta, mascarpone is a great alternative to traditional cream cheese, as it's lower in fat and contains almost no sodium.

1. Preheat oven to 350°F. Take out a 12-inch pizza pan and set aside.

2. In a mixing bowl, cream together the butter and sugar.

3. Add the vanilla, lemon juice, and lemon zest and mix well.

4. Gradually add in the flour, alternating with the milk.

5. Remove dough from bowl and roll out to a (roughly) 12-inch circle. Transfer dough to pan and gently press into the bottom.

6. Place pan on middle rack in oven and bake for 15 minutes. Remove from oven and set on wire rack to cool to room temperature.

7. While crust is cooling, prepare the topping. Beat together the mascarpone, sour cream, and powdered sugar.

8. When the crust is cool, spread evenly over surface. Decorate as desired with sliced fresh fruit.

9. Serve immediately or cover and refrigerate until serving. Best eaten within a day of baking.

PER SERVING | Calories: 228 | Fat: 7 g | Protein: 3 g | Sodium: 36 mg | Fiber: 1 g | Carbohydrates: 38 g | Sugar: 19 g

Peppermint Watermelon Granita

Delightfully tingly, this refreshing dessert is the perfect end to a summer meal.
Garnish with fresh mint leaves and extra cubed watermelon if desired.

INGREDIENTS | SERVES 6

3 peppermint tea bags
3 cups boiling water
3 cups fresh watermelon, cubed
1 tablespoon agave nectar

Watermelon Facts

Watermelon is closely related to ground melons and squash. It's low in fat, a good source of fiber, and as its name suggests, one of the juiciest fruits around. Watermelon contains high levels of vitamins A and C as well as lycopene, a cancer-fighting antioxidant. To select a perfectly ripe watermelon, hold it close to your body and thump firmly. If it sounds and feels hollow, it's a keeper. Put back any without reverb; they tend to be mealy.

1. Place tea bags in a heatproof pitcher or tea pot. Add boiling water and steep 5 minutes.

2. Place cubed watermelon into a blender or food processor and purée.

3. Remove tea bags and pour liquid into a 9" × 13" freezer-safe pan.

4. Add watermelon and agave and stir to combine. Cover pan and place in freezer.

5. Freeze 2–3 hours. Remove from freezer and scrape mixture into glasses or bowls. Serve immediately.

PER SERVING | Calories: 32 | Fat: 0 g | Protein: 0 g | Sodium: 0 mg | Fiber: 0 g | Carbohydrates: 8 g | Sugar: 7 g

Guilt-Free Chocolate Cupcakes

Whole-grain cupcakes that are truly good for you. Low fat, low sodium, and vegan, too. Indulge in moist, dense, chocolate-laden pleasure with absolutely no guilt!

INGREDIENTS | YIELDS 16

1⅔ cups white whole-wheat flour
¾ cup light brown sugar
¼ cup unsweetened cocoa powder
2 teaspoons sodium-free baking soda
1 cup water
½ cup unsweetened applesauce
1 teaspoon pure vanilla extract
½ cup semisweet chocolate chips

1. Preheat oven to 350°F. Line 2 muffin tins with paper liners and set aside.

2. Place the dry ingredients, except chocolate chips, into a mixing bowl and whisk together.

3. Add the wet ingredients to the pan and mix until combined.

4. Pour batter into the muffin cups, filing rough ⅔ full.

5. Sprinkle chocolate chips evenly over the batter.

6. Place pan on middle rack in oven and bake for 20 minutes. Remove from oven and place on wire rack to cool. Cool briefly before serving.

PER SERVING | Calories: 123 | Fat: 2 g | Protein: 2 g | Sodium: 4 mg | Fiber: 2 g | Carbohydrates: 25 g | Sugar: 15 g

Best Low-Sodium Birthday Cake

Everyone deserves a special treat on their big day. This cake combines the best of both worlds, producing an ultra moist, absolutely delicious cake, while keeping health in mind. The recipe yields 1 (8-inch) layer cake, a 9" × 13" pan, or 24 cupcakes.

INGREDIENTS | SERVES 12

2¾ cups cake flour

1½ cups sugar

1 tablespoon sodium-free baking powder

3 egg whites

⅔ cup vegetable oil

1 cup low-fat milk

1 tablespoon pure vanilla extract

2 teaspoons pure almond extract

Frosting

4 tablespoons unsalted butter

3 cups powdered sugar

3 tablespoons low-fat milk

2 teaspoons pure vanilla extract

2 tablespoons unsweetened cocoa powder

Easy Greasing

The simplest way to grease and flour a pan is by using an oil cooking spray. Spray pan lightly with oil, add a tablespoon of flour, then tap pan and invert to disperse. After surface is evenly coated, tip pan over the sink, compost bin, or trash can and tap lightly to remove excess flour.

1. Preheat oven to 350°F. Grease and flour 2 (8-inch) round pans and set aside.

2. Place the flour, sugar, and baking powder into a large mixing bowl and whisk well to combine.

3. Add the egg whites, oil, milk, and extracts and beat for 2 minutes.

4. Pour batter into prepared pans, dividing evenly, and place on middle rack in oven. Bake for 25 minutes for 2 (8-inch) pans or 1 (9" × 13") pan, or for 20 minutes for 24 cupcakes.

5. Remove from oven and set on wire rack to cool. Cool briefly before carefully removing layer cakes from pans. Cool fully before frosting.

6. To make the frosting, place the butter into a mixing bowl.

7. Gradually add in the powdered sugar, beating well.

8. Add the milk, vanilla, and cocoa and beat until combined. Frost cake as desired.

PER SERVING (CAKE AND FROSTING) | Calories: 486 | Fat: 16 g | Protein: 4 g | Sodium: 26 mg | Fiber: 1 g | Carbohydrates: 81 g | Sugar: 55 g

Pound Cake Minis

Save these rich little cakes for a seriously special occasion.
Although healthier than classic pound cake, they're still pretty decadent.

INGREDIENTS | YIELDS 18

½ cup unsalted butter

¼ cup nonhydrogenated vegetable shortening

1 cup sugar

2 egg whites

2 teaspoons pure vanilla extract

¼ teaspoon pure almond extract

½ teaspoon sodium-free baking powder

1¼ cups unbleached all-purpose flour

½ cup low-fat milk

1. Preheat oven to 350°F. Line 18 muffin cups with paper liners and set aside.

2. Place the butter and shortening into a mixing bowl.

3. Add the sugar and beat until fluffy.

4. Beat in the egg whites and extracts.

5. Stir in the baking powder and gradually add in the flour, alternating with the milk, and stir until combined.

6. Spoon batter into muffin tins, filling each cup about ⅔ full. Place muffin tins on middle rack in oven and bake for 20 minutes.

7. Remove from oven and transfer to a wire rack to cool.

PER SERVING | Calories: 150 | Fat: 8 g | Protein: 1 g | Sodium: 10 mg | Fiber: 0 g | Carbohydrates: 18 g | Sugar: 11 g

Karen's Apple Kugel

A healthy dessert that also makes a great side dish or breakfast. The softened matzo gives this kugel a creamy texture and appearance without adding additional fat, cholesterol, or sodium. Many thanks to friend and Daily Dish reader, Karen, for sharing!

INGREDIENTS | SERVES 8

3 sheets unsalted matzo

2 cups water

4 tart green apples

1 tablespoon freshly squeezed lemon juice

3 tablespoons unsalted butter, melted

¼ cup brown sugar

½ cup seedless raisins

3 egg whites

1½ teaspoons ground cinnamon

What Is Matzo?

Matzo is a type of unleavened bread, traditionally composed of only flour and water. Although associated with the Jewish Passover holiday, matzo can be purchased year round in most places, and is typically stocked in the kosher section of the supermarket. Matzo have a large cracker-like appearance and often contain little to no sodium, making them a terrific base for peanut butter and jelly sandwiches, Swiss cheese, hummus, and more.

1. Preheat oven to 350°F. Take out an 8" × 11" baking dish and set aside.

2. Place the matzo in an 8-inch square baking pan. Pour the water into the pan and set aside to rehydrate.

3. Peel apples, core, and cut into quarters. Cut each quarter crosswise into thirds, and lengthwise into slices no more than ¼-inch thick. Transfer apples to a mixing bowl.

4. Check on the matzo. When soft, drain the matzo and squeeze out excess water.

5. Place matzo into the mixing bowl. Add the remaining ingredients and stir well to combine.

6. Pour mixture into the 8" × 11" baking dish. Place dish on middle rack in oven and bake for 30 minutes.

7. Remove from oven. Set on a wire rack to cool. Cut into portions and serve warm or cool.

PER SERVING | Calories: 181 | Fat: 4 g | Protein: 3 g | Sodium: 24 mg | Fiber: 2 g | Carbohydrates: 34 g | Sugar: 21 g

Vegan Rice Pudding

This recipe produces a delicious nondairy rice pudding that's thick and creamy, with just a hint of the exotic. The pudding thickens significantly as it cools; if you prefer a thinner consistency, stir in a little nondairy milk before serving.

INGREDIENTS | SERVES 8

1 quart vanilla nondairy milk
1 cup basmati or jasmine rice, rinsed
¼ cup sugar
1 teaspoon pure vanilla extract
⅛ teaspoon pure almond extract
½ teaspoon ground cinnamon
⅛ teaspoon ground cardamom

1. Measure all of the ingredients into a saucepan and stir well to combine. Bring to a boil over medium-high heat.

2. Once boiling, reduce heat to low and simmer, stirring very frequently, about 15–20 minutes.

3. Remove from heat and cool. Serve sprinkled with ground cinnamon if desired.

PER SERVING | Calories: 148 | Fat: 2 g | Protein: 4 g | Sodium: 48 mg | Fiber: 1 g | Carbohydrates: 26 g | Sugar: 10 g

Homemade Banana Ice Cream

This dessert contains only one ingredient: bananas. Yet when frozen and puréed, the crystallized fruit mimics the look, taste, and texture of ice cream so perfectly, it's almost magic.

INGREDIENTS | SERVES 4

4 ripe bananas

1. Place unpeeled bananas in freezer and freeze until solid.

2. Remove bananas from freezer, peel, and slice into chunks. Place chunks into a blender or food processor and pulse until smooth.

3. Scoop mixture out and serve immediately.

PER SERVING | Calories: 105 | Fat: 0 g | Protein: 1 g | Sodium: 1 mg | Fiber: 3 g | Carbohydrates: 26 g | Sugar: 14 g

Instant Chocolate Pudding

Sweet, luscious, and absolutely divine, this pudding whips together in mere minutes. If you don't disclose it's vegan, no one will ever know. Bring the tofu to room temperature before assembly; you want the chocolate to stay fluid and not seize up.

INGREDIENTS | SERVES 4

¾ cup semisweet chocolate chips

1 pound silken tofu, at room temperature

¼ cup sugar

½ teaspoon pure vanilla extract

Silken Tofu

The soft, smooth texture of silken tofu makes it a great stand-in for eggs and dairy in many recipes. Silken tofu adds protein and creaminess while being cholesterol and sodium free. It's also low in fat, and its bland taste allows other ingredients to shine. Use silken tofu instead of milk when making smoothies and puddings, or try adding it in lieu of sour cream or yogurt in your favorite dips and dressings.

1. To melt chocolate in the microwave, place in a microwave-safe bowl and heat on high for 45 seconds. Remove and stir until smooth. To melt on the stovetop, place in a small saucepan over low heat and stir until melted.

2. Place the tofu in a food processor and pulse until smooth.

3. Add the melted chocolate, sugar, and vanilla and pulse to combine.

4. Serve immediately or cover and refrigerate until ready to serve.

PER SERVING | Calories: 329 | Fat: 16 g | Protein: 10 g | Sodium: 9 mg | Fiber: 3 g | Carbohydrates: 44 g | Sugar: 37 g

Blueberry Pudding Cake

Luscious berries oozing into a soft, semisolid cake.
This homey dessert is heaven in a bowl.

INGREDIENTS | SERVES 6

3 cups fresh ripe blueberries

¾ cup sugar, divided

1 tablespoon freshly squeezed lemon juice

6 tablespoons unsalted butter, softened

2 teaspoons pure vanilla extract

1 teaspoon freshly grated lemon zest

1 egg white

1½ teaspoons sodium-free baking powder

2 tablespoons low-fat milk

⅔ cup unbleached all-purpose flour

Blueberry Facts

Blueberries have been harvested for thousands of years in North America, and are an easy garden crop, requiring only acidic soil and adequate rainfall. Blueberries are high in vitamins K and C as well as manganese, and contain several antioxidants believed to inhibit cancer and inflammation. Fresh blueberries make a delicious addition to baked goods, salads, and sauces, but when fresh are fairly perishable. To prevent spoilage, freeze blueberries and thaw as needed.

1. Preheat oven to 375°F. Spray an 8-inch square baking pan lightly with oil and set aside.

2. Place blueberries into a mixing bowl. Add ¼ cup sugar and lemon juice and toss well to coat.

3. Pour berries into the baking dish, place on middle rack in oven, and bake for 10 minutes. Remove from oven and set aside.

4. Place the butter and remaining ½ cup sugar into a mixing bowl and beat to combine.

5. Add the vanilla, lemon zest, and egg white and mix well.

6. Add the baking powder and milk and stir. Gradually add in the flour, mixing until combined.

7. Pour batter over the cooked blueberries. Place pan on middle rack in oven and bake for 20 minutes, until golden brown.

8. Remove from oven and place pan on wire rack to cool. Serve warm or cool.

PER SERVING | Calories: 300 | Fat: 12 g | Protein: 2 g | Sodium: 14 mg | Fiber: 2 g | Carbohydrates: 46 g | Sugar: 32 g

Peach Cobbler

An updated version of the classic dessert with heart-healthy whole grain and ripe juicy fruit. Serve with whipped cream and/or nonfat frozen yogurt if desired.

INGREDIENTS | SERVES 8

6 ripe peaches, peeled and sliced

3 tablespoons sugar

Juice of 1 fresh lemon

1¼ cups unbleached all-purpose flour

½ cup white whole-wheat flour

⅔ cup sugar

1 teaspoon sodium-free baking powder

4 tablespoons unsalted butter, melted and cooled

1 egg white

½ cup low-fat milk

1 tablespoon pure vanilla extract

1. Preheat oven to 400°F. Get out a 9" × 13" baking dish and set aside.

2. Place sliced peaches into a mixing bowl, add sugar and lemon juice, and toss well to coat. Transfer to the baking dish. Set aside.

3. Measure the flours, sugar, and baking powder into a mixing bowl and whisk well to combine.

4. Add the melted butter, egg white, milk, and vanilla and stir well to combine. Batter will be thick. Spoon batter over sliced peaches.

5. Place pan on middle rack in oven and bake for 30 minutes.

6. Remove pan from oven and place on wire rack to cool. Serve warm or cool.

PER SERVING | Calories: 273 | Fat: 6 g | Protein: 5 g | Sodium: 15 mg | Fiber: 3 g | Carbohydrates: 50 g | Sugar: 28 g

Sautéed Bananas

This dessert is truly divine. Fabulous on its own or spooned over nonfat frozen yogurt. So simple and so good.

INGREDIENTS | SERVES 2

1½ tablespoons unsalted butter

¼ cup brown sugar

½ teaspoon pure vanilla extract

1 tablespoon low-fat milk

2 large ripe bananas, cut into chunks

1 tablespoon chopped walnuts

Walnut Facts

Walnuts have a wonderfully nutty flavor that complements almost everything from baked goods to side dishes, salads, and entrées. They're rich in monounsaturated fats and omega-3 fatty acids, manganese, and copper, and have been shown to prevent cardiovascular disease, lower cholesterol, and inhibit certain types of cancer.

1. Melt butter in a skillet over medium-high.

2. Once melted, add the brown sugar, vanilla, and milk and stir until sugar has dissolved and a thick syrup forms, about 30 seconds.

3. Add the bananas, tilt pan slightly so that the syrup slides to the bottom, then spoon syrup over banana continuously, warming the slices and basting 2–3 minutes.

4. Remove from heat and serve immediately, garnished with chopped walnuts.

PER SERVING | Calories: 312 | Fat: 10 g | Protein: 2 g | Sodium: 14 mg | Fiber: 3 g | Carbohydrates: 58 g | Sugar: 43 g

Strawberry Shortcake

The second-best way to serve gorgeous, ripe, red strawberries, topped only by eating them plain. Add a scoop of nonfat frozen yogurt to make sundaes. Light whipped cream is sold in aerated cans in the refrigerated dairy case of most supermarkets.

INGREDIENTS | SERVES 4

4 Baking Powder Biscuits (see Chapter 3)
1 pound ripe strawberries, sliced
2 tablespoons sugar
1 cup light whipped cream

1. Slice biscuits in half. Place the bottom of each into a serving bowl and set the tops aside.

2. Place sliced strawberries in a mixing bowl, sprinkle sugar over top, and stir to coat. Let sit several minutes to release juice.

3. Spoon berries over the biscuit bottoms, then cover with the tops. Spoon excess syrup over top of the biscuits, then garnish with whipped cream. Serve immediately.

PER SERVING | Calories: 265 | Fat: 14 g | Protein: 4 g | Sodium: 24 mg | Fiber: 3 g | Carbohydrates: 32 g | Sugar: 12 g

Baked Apple Slices

Apple pie without the fattening crust. These slices make a delicious dessert served plain or over ice cream, a scrumptious topping for pancakes, even a tasty side for dinner. Talk about versatile!

INGREDIENTS | SERVES 4

6 medium apples, sliced
2 tablespoons unsalted butter, melted
¼ cup light brown sugar
1 teaspoon ground cinnamon

1. Preheat oven to 450°F.

2. Place apples, butter, brown sugar, and cinnamon into a mixing bowl and toss well to coat.

3. Transfer to a shallow baking dish and cover tightly with foil. Place dish on middle rack in oven and bake for 20 minutes.

4. Remove from oven, carefully remove foil, and stir gently to recoat apples with sauce. Serve immediately.

PER SERVING | Calories: 244 | Fat: 6 g | Protein: <1 g | Sodium: 7 mg | Fiber: 6 g | Carbohydrates: 51 g | Sugar: 41 g

Tracie's Whoopie Pies

Whoopie pies aren't exactly health food, but as an occasional treat these are perfect. This version is lower in fat, cholesterol, and calories than the standard variety, and adds healthy whole-grain flour to the mix. Many thanks to Tracie for sharing!

INGREDIENTS | YIELDS 9

1½ cups unbleached all-purpose flour
½ cup white whole-wheat flour
¾ cup sugar
⅓ cup unsweetened cocoa powder
2 teaspoons sodium-free baking soda
1 egg white
⅓ cup canola oil
¾ cup low-fat milk
4 tablespoons unsalted butter
2 teaspoons pure vanilla extract
6 tablespoons marshmallow fluff
2 cups powdered sugar

Desserts and Diet

People often equate dieting with deprivation, but sweets can be part of a healthy lifestyle when chosen wisely and consumed in moderation. If you're someone with an above-average sweet tooth, try to channel cravings into the healthy realm of fruit. Keep an array of fresh produce out on the counter and you'll find yourself reaching for it daily. Dried fruit, applesauce, and juice-sweetened fruit cups also make great guilt-free treats.

1. Preheat oven to 375°F. Line a large baking sheet with parchment and set aside.

2. Place the flours, sugar, cocoa powder, and baking soda into a mixing bowl and whisk to combine.

3. Add the egg white, oil, and milk and beat well.

4. Drop by heaping tablespoonfuls onto the prepared baking sheet. Place sheet on middle rack in oven and bake for 10 minutes.

5. Remove sheet from oven. Remove cookie halves from baking sheet and transfer to a wire rack to cool. Repeat process with remaining batter.

6. Melt the butter in a saucepan over medium heat. Once melted, remove from heat, add the remaining ingredients, and stir well to combine. If frosting is too dry, add a tiny bit of low-fat milk and beat until smooth.

7. Once the cookie halves have cooled, make sandwiches out of them by spreading filling on one half and sandwiching with another. Store in an airtight container or wrap in plastic.

PER SERVING | Calories: 408 | Fat: 14 g | Protein: 4 g | Sodium: 19 mg | Fiber: 2 g | Carbohydrates: 68 g | Sugar: 45 g

Plum Cake

*An absolutely amazing dessert! Juicy slices of plum soften in the oven,
sinking into a moist almond-flavored cake. Substitute other fresh fruit if desired.*

INGREDIENTS | SERVES 12

3 medium plums
Egg replacement powder for 2 eggs
1 cup unbleached all-purpose flour
¼ cup white whole-wheat flour
⅔ cup sugar
2 teaspoons sodium-free baking powder
1 teaspoon pure almond extract
1 teaspoon pure vanilla extract
⅓ cup canola oil
½ cup vanilla nondairy milk

Plum Facts

Plums are a stone fruit, similar to nectarines and peaches, and contain high levels of vitamins A, C, K, and fiber. Their light, sweet taste complements many salads, side dishes, and desserts. Dried plums, also known as prunes, have a concentrated sweetness that can be enjoyed on its own or used in lieu of sugar. Soak prunes in hot water, then purée and add to baked goods, oatmeal, or other hot cereals.

1. Preheat oven to 375°F. Grease and flour an 8" × 11" baking pan and set aside.

2. Slice plums in half and remove pits. Slice each half into quarters and set aside.

3. Prepare egg replacement powder according to package directions. Set aside.

4. Place the flours, sugar, and baking powder into a mixing bowl and whisk well to combine.

5. Add the egg replacement, extracts, oil, and milk and stir well to combine.

6. Spread batter evenly in the prepared pan, then arrange plum slices neatly over top. Place pan on middle rack in oven and bake for 30 minutes.

7. Remove from oven and place pan on a wire rack to cool. Serve warm or cool.

PER SERVING | Calories: 175 | Fat: 7 g | Protein: 4 g | Sodium: 38 mg | Fiber: 1 g | Carbohydrates: 24 g | Sugar: 14 g